TYPE 2 DIABETES
DIET COOKBOOK

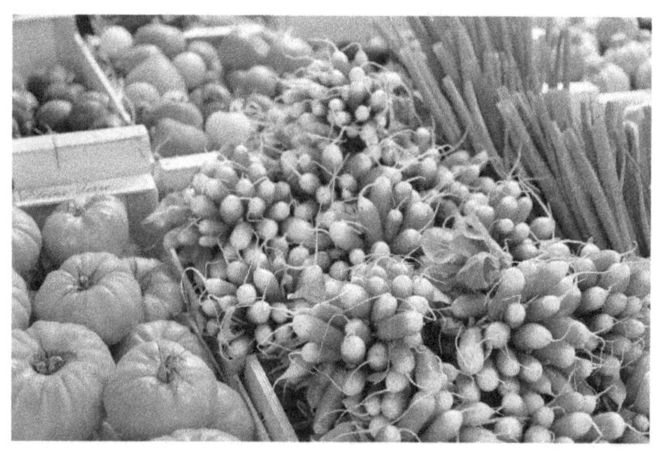

1800 Days of Nourishing Wellness with Delectable Low Carbs and Low Sugar Recipes

Angela W. Ashley

TABLE OF CONTENT

INTRODUCTION

In the bustling city, where fast-paced lifestyles frequently influenced nutritional choices, a silent revolution was taking place in kitchens across the neighborhood. It all started with a group of friends who were dealing with the same problem: Type 2 diabetes. Determined to take control of their health, they set out on a trip that would not only change their lives but also inspire others to follow suit. The movement was led by a seasoned chef.

Amidst a sea of fad diets and conflicting nutrition advice, she urged the group to take a more holistic and long-term strategy to controlling their disease. The reason for change was a shared love of cooking and a desire to produce meals that were both delicious and diabetic-friendly. So, the idea of creating a cookbook exclusively for those with Type 2 diabetes was born. The cookbook, appropriately titled "TYPE 2 DIABETES COOKBOOK," is more than simply a compilation of dishes; it's a story about resilience, friendship, and the victory of adopting a healthy lifestyle. Each page is a story of discovery, from navigating grocery store aisles to deciphering food labels. The author walks readers through the complexities of mindful eating.

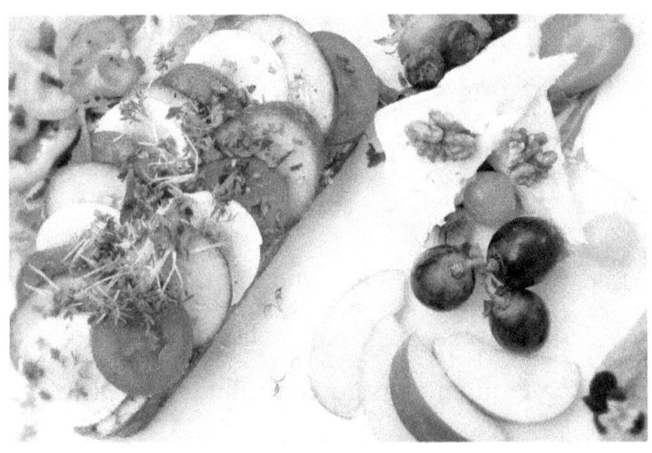

The introduction to "TYPE 2 DIABETES COOKBOOK" dives into the author's own experiences. She openly discusses their initial shock at their diagnosis, the difficulties of adjusting to new food limitations, and their shared commitment to transform their kitchens into sanctuaries of well-being. Readers engage with the human side of diabetes management through anecdotes and thoughts, taking comfort in these individuals' shared difficulties and achievements. The introduction also serves as an educational tool, explaining the complexity of Type 2 diabetes. It presents a quick but comprehensive description of the illness, emphasizing the role of diet in its treatment.

As the story progresses, the author incorporates the science behind the recipes, describing how each dish is thoughtfully designed to adhere to diabetes-friendly principles. From conscious carbohydrate choices to the strategic use of herbs and spices, the cookbook serves as a culinary guide, providing readers with the skills they need to make informed and delicious decisions in their own kitchens.

"TYPE 2 DIABETES COOKBOOK" is more than just a set of recipes; it's a genuine invitation to start on a transforming culinary journey. It lays the groundwork for a cookbook that goes beyond the confines of a medical condition, telling a story of optimism, companionship, and the joy of savoring every balanced bite on the path to a better future.

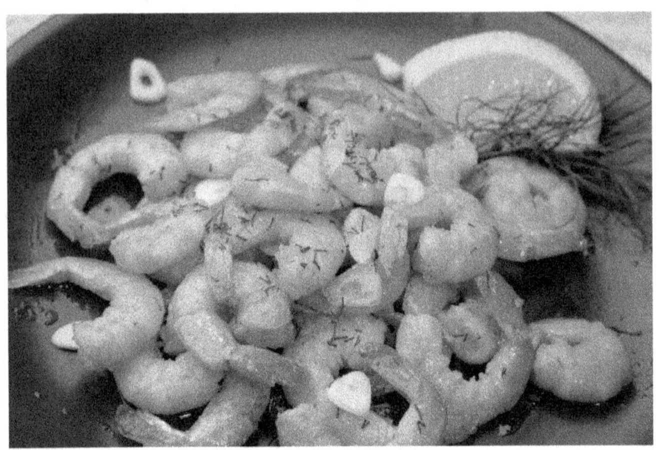

CHAPTER 1:

UNDERSTANDING TYPE 2

DIABETES (T2D)

What is Type 2 Diabetes?

Type 2 diabetes (T2D) is a chronic metabolic condition characterized by high blood sugar levels due to insulin resistance and insufficient insulin synthesis. In this situation, cells do not respond properly to insulin, a hormone required for glucose absorption. Over time, the pancreas, which is responsible for insulin secretion, may become less efficient. It is most common among adults, but it can afflict people of any age. Lifestyle changes, medicines, and, on occasion, insulin therapy are used to manage the condition. Complications may include heart disease, kidney problems, and nerve damage.

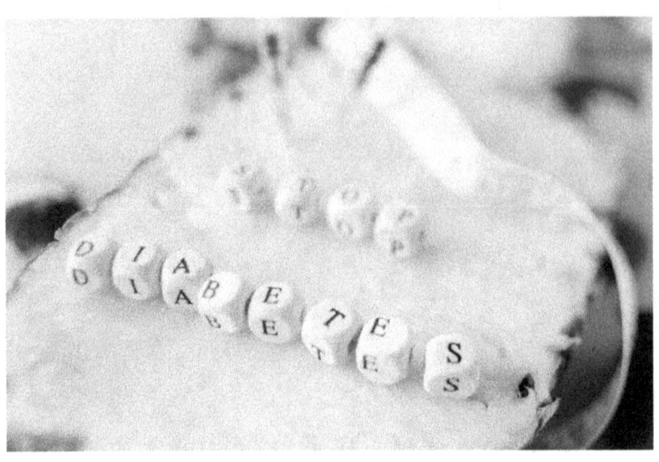

What are the possible causes?

- Patients with the family history of type 2 diabetes is at a higher risk of having it.

- Lifestyle factors like poor diet, inactivity, and obesity can also increase the chances of having type 2 diabetes.

- The risk of having type 2 diabetes rises with age, particularly after 45.

- Conditions like high blood pressure and abnormal cholesterol levels can also cause it.

- Poor sleep can reduce insulin sensitivity.

- Women commonly have polycystic ovarian syndrome (PCOS), which is associated with insulin resistance.

- A sedentary lifestyle increases diabetes risk.

- <u>Ethnicity</u>: Certain ethnic groups have a higher risk for type 2 diabetes.

- <u>Insulin resistance</u>: Cells do not respond well to insulin.

Can proper diet help manage Type 2 Diabetes?

- A well-balanced diet helps regulate blood glucose levels, minimizing surges and ensuring stability in those with type 2 diabetes.

- Carbohydrate consumption must be monitored and controlled since carbs have a direct impact on blood sugar levels.

- Fiber-rich meals, such as whole grains and vegetables, aid digestion and improve blood sugar control.

- Consuming lean proteins helps to retain muscle mass, offers continuous energy, and prevents excessive consumption of saturated fats.

- Unsaturated fats, such as those found in avocados and almonds, promote heart health and help reduce cholesterol levels.

- Staying hydrated improves overall health and can help lower blood sugar levels.

- Limiting portion sizes helps to manage calorie intake, promotes weight management, and prevents insulin resistance.

- Meal timing is important for regulating insulin response and maintaining stable blood sugar levels.

- Tailoring dietary regimens to individual needs and preferences lead to improved adherence and long-term effectiveness in diabetes control.

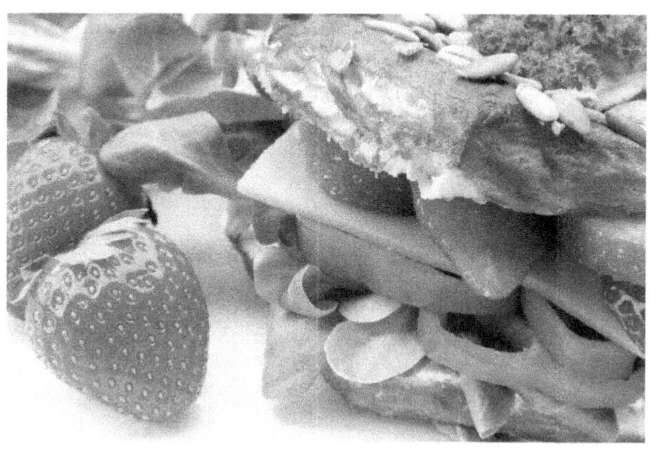

Food choices that can help manage Type 2 Diabetes

Here are some meal options appropriate for those with type 2 diabetes:

- Non-Starchy vegetables like broccoli, spinach, cauliflower, bell peppers and so on.
- Whole Grains like quinoa. v\brown rice, oats and so on.
- Lean Proteins: Skinless poultry, fish, tofu and legumes.
- Healthy Fats: avocado, olive oil, nuts.

- Low-Fat Dairy: cottage cheese, Greek yogurt.

- Fruits like berries, apples, pears.

- Limit or avoid sugary beverages, fried foods, refined grains and so on.

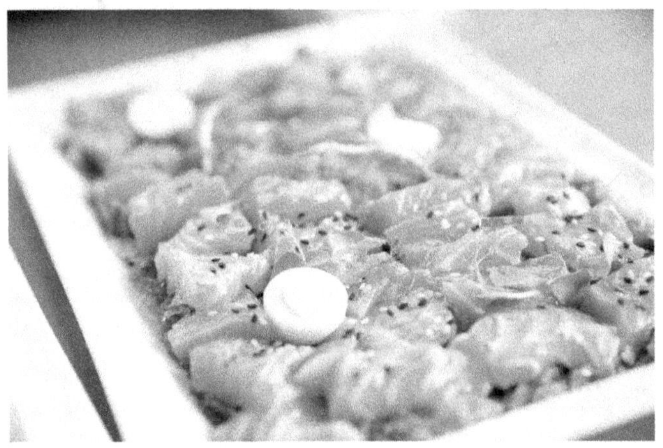

Frequently Asked Questions

Can the recipes in this cookbook help me regulate my blood sugar effectively? Yes, the recipes are intended to include balanced nutrients that promote stable blood sugar control in those with type 2 diabetes.

What role may these dishes play in type 2 diabetes weight management? The cookbook emphasizes portion control, nutrient balance, and whole, unprocessed foods to aid with weight management as part of a diabetes-friendly lifestyle.

Can the entire family, including non-diabetics, appreciate these recipes? Yes, the recipes are designed to be enjoyable and suited for the entire family, encouraging a balanced and health-conscious way of eating.

Are there any options for vegans or others with dietary restrictions? Yes, the cookbook has a variety of recipes catering to various food needs, including vegetarian options and those with dietary restrictions.

Are the ingredients in the recipes easily available at local grocery stores? Yes, the cookbook stresses commonly available and popular ingredients to enable convenience and accessibility for all.

How can I customize these recipes to suit my specific taste preferences? The cookbook promotes experimentation and offers modification advice, allowing you to tailor flavors and ingredients to your specific preferences while adhering to diabetes-friendly principles.

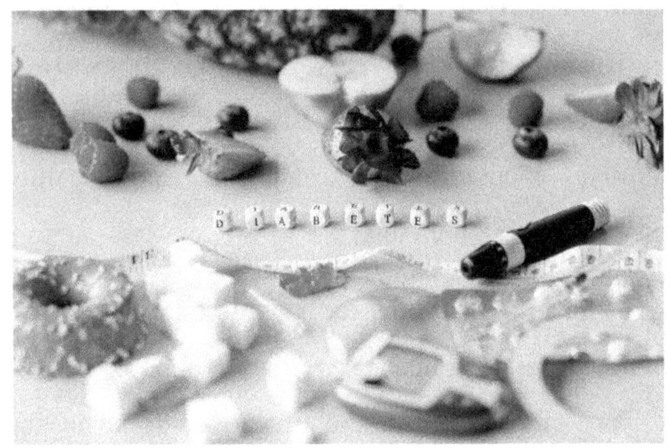

CHAPTER 2: BREAKFAST RECIPES

Veggie Omelet:

Ingredients:

- Eggs
- Diced bell peppers
- Spinach
- Cherry tomatoes

Instructions:

- Whisk the eggs and pour into a hot, non-stick pan.
- Add the vegetables and simmer until the eggs are set.

Prep Time: 10 minutes

Nutritional Information: Protein, calories, carbs and fiber

Greek Yogurt Parfait:

Ingredients:

- Greek yogurt
- Mixed berries
- Chopped nuts
- Honey (optional)

<u>Instructions</u>:

- Layer yogurt, berries, and nuts in a glass.
- Drizzle with honey if preferred.

<u>Prep Time</u>: 5 minutes

<u>Nutritional Information</u>: Protein, calories, carbs and fiber

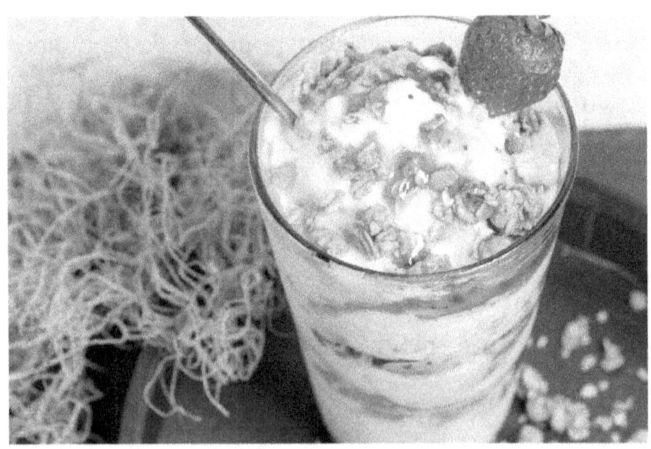

Quinoa Breakfast Bowl:

Ingredients:

- Cooked quinoa

- Almond milk

- Diced mango

- Chia seeds

Instructions:

- Mix the quinoa with almond milk.

- Add mango and chia seeds as toppings.

Prep Time: 15 minutes

Nutritional Information: Protein, calories, carbs and fiber

Whole Grain Toast with Avocado:

Ingredients:

- Slices of whole-grain bread

- Mashed Avocado

- Olive oil

- Salt and pepper

<u>Instructions</u>:

- Toast the bread slices.
- Spread the mashed avocado on the toasted bread slices
- Drizzle with olive oil, then season.

<u>Prep Time</u>: 8 minutes

<u>Nutritional Information</u>: Protein, calories, carbs and fiber

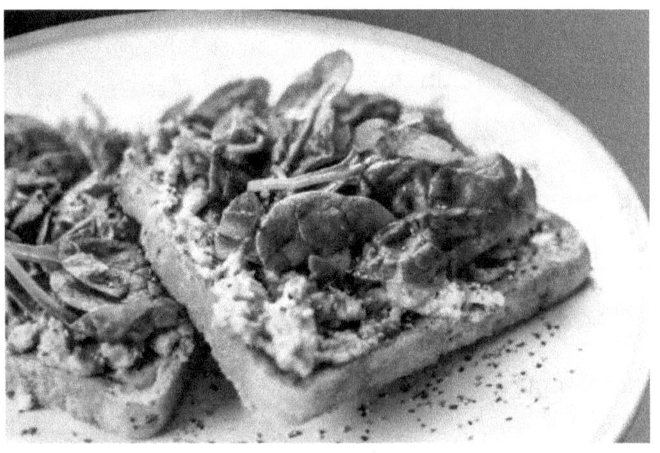

Cottage Cheese and Berry Bowl:

<u>Ingredients</u>:

- Cottage cheese

- Mixed berries

- Flaxseeds

- Vanilla extract

<u>Instructions</u>:

- Mix the cottage cheese with berries, flaxseeds, and vanilla.

- Mix thoroughly and serve.

<u>Prep Time</u>: 7 minutes

<u>Nutritional Information</u>: Protein, calories, carbs and fiber

Spinach and Mushroom Frittata:

<u>Ingredients</u>:

- Eggs
- Spinach
- Mushrooms
- Feta cheese

<u>Instructions</u>:

- Sauté mushrooms and spinach.

- Pour the whisked eggs over it.

- Add the feta and bake until the mixture is set.

Prep Time: 25 minutes

Nutritional Information: Packed with vitamins and protein.

Chia Seed Pudding:

Ingredients:

- Chia seeds
- Unsweetened almond milk
- Vanilla extract

Instructions:

- Mix the ingredients together.
- Refrigerate overnight.
- Add berries as toppings.

Prep Time: 5 minutes (plus overnight soaking)

Nutritional Information: Fiber and omega-3 fatty acids

Turkey and Veggie Breakfast Burrito:

Ingredients:

- Whole-grain tortilla
- Lean ground turkey
- Bell peppers
- Onions

Instructions:

- Sauté the turkey and vegetables.
- Fill and wrap the tortilla.

Prep Time: 15 minutes

Nutritional Information: Protein and fiber

Oatmeal with Berries and Nuts:

Ingredients:

- Rolled oats
- Almond milk
- Mixed berries
- Almonds

<u>Instructions:</u>

- Cook the oats.

- Add the berries and almonds as toppings.

<u>Prep Time</u>: 10 minutes

<u>Nutritional Information</u>: High in fiber and antioxidants

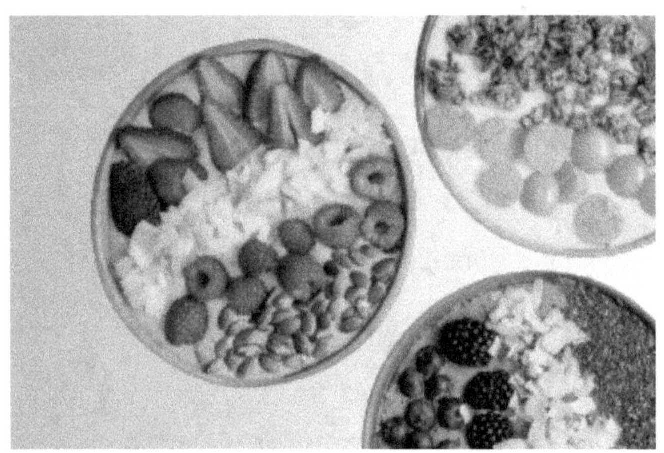

Low-Carb Smoothie:

<u>Ingredients:</u>

- Unsweetened almond milk

- Spinach

- Cucumber

- Chia seeds
- Protein powder

Instructions:

- Blend all the ingredients together until smooth.
- Serve and enjoy.

Prep Time: 5 minutes

Nutritional Information: Low in carbs, rich in nutrients

Almond Flour Pancakes:

Ingredients:

- Almond flour
- Eggs
- Almond milk
- Baking powder

Instructions:

- Mix the ingredients together.
- Make small pancakes and serve with sugar-free syrup.

<u>Prep Time</u>: 15 minutes

<u>Nutritional Information</u>: Low in carbs, high in protein

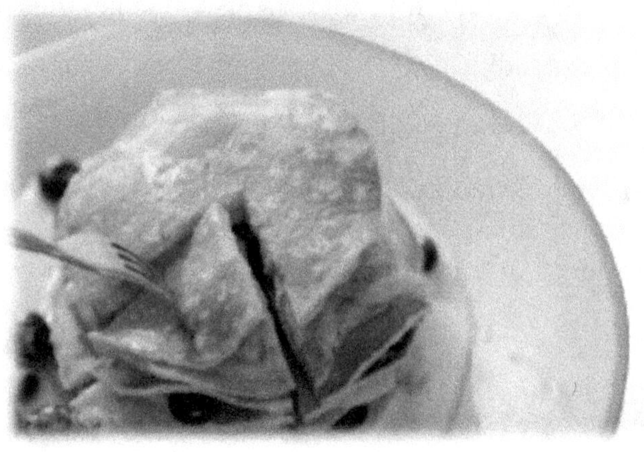

Smoked Salmon and Cream Cheese Bagel:

<u>Ingredients</u>:

- Whole-grain bagel
- Smoked salmon
- Light cream cheese

<u>Instructions</u>:

- Toast the bagels.

- Spread the cream cheese, then top with the smoked salmon.

Prep Time: 10 minutes

Nutritional Information: Omega-3 fatty acids and protein

Mediterranean Breakfast Bowl:

Ingredients:

- Quinoa
- Cherry tomatoes
- Cucumber
- Olives
- Feta cheese

Instructions:

- Layer the ingredients in a bowl.
- Serve and enjoy!

Prep Time: 20 minutes

Nutritional Information: Healthy fats

Egg and Veggie Breakfast Wrap:

<u>Ingredients</u>:

- Whole-grain wrap
- Scrambled eggs
- Bell peppers
- Onions
- Salsa

<u>Instructions</u>:

- Fill the wrap with eggs, sautéed veggies, and salsa.
- Serve and enjoy.

<u>Prep Time</u>: 15 minutes

<u>Nutritional Information</u>: Rich in fiber and protein

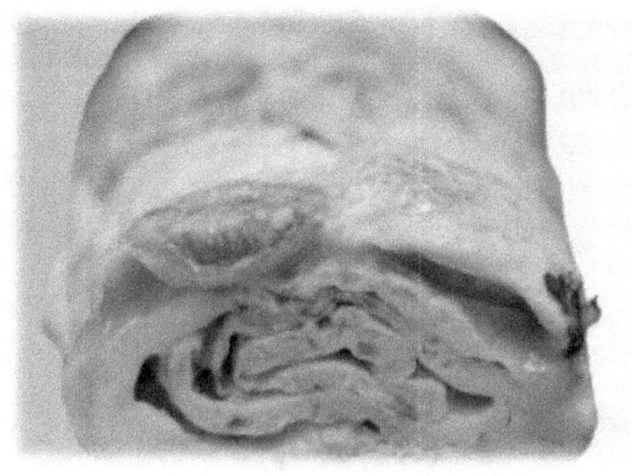

Yogurt and Berry Smoothie Bowl:

<u>Ingredients</u>:

- Greek yogurt
- Mixed berries
- Granola

<u>Instructions</u>:

- Blend the yogurt with mixed berries.
- Pour the mixture into a bowl and top with berries and granola.

<u>Prep Time</u>: 10 minutes

: Protein, fiber, and antioxidants

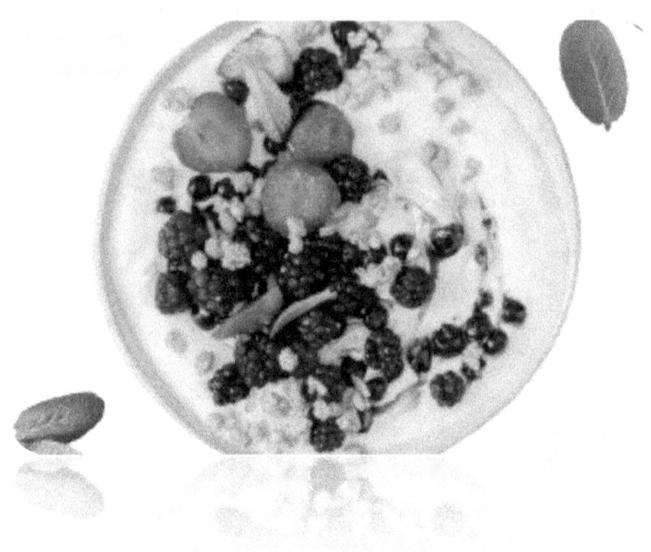

Cauliflower Hash Browns:

Ingredients:

- Grated cauliflower
- Eggs
- Onion
- Garlic powder

Instructions:

- Mix the ingredients together.
- Form patties and cook until golden brown.

<u>Prep Time</u>: 20 minutes

<u>Nutritional Information</u>: Vitamins

Peanut Butter Banana Toast:

<u>Ingredients</u>:

- Whole-grain bread
- Natural peanut butter
- Banana slices

<u>Instructions</u>:

- Toast the bread.
- Add peanut butter and top with banana slices.

<u>Prep Time</u>: 5 minutes

<u>Nutritional Information</u>: Healthy fats and potassium

Tomato and Basil Avocado Toast:

<u>Ingredients</u>:

- Whole-grain bread

- Avocado

- Cherry tomatoes

- Fresh basil

Instructions:

- Mash the avocado.

- Put it on the toast, and top with tomatoes and basil.

Prep Time: 10 minutes

Nutritional Information: Vitamins and healthy fats

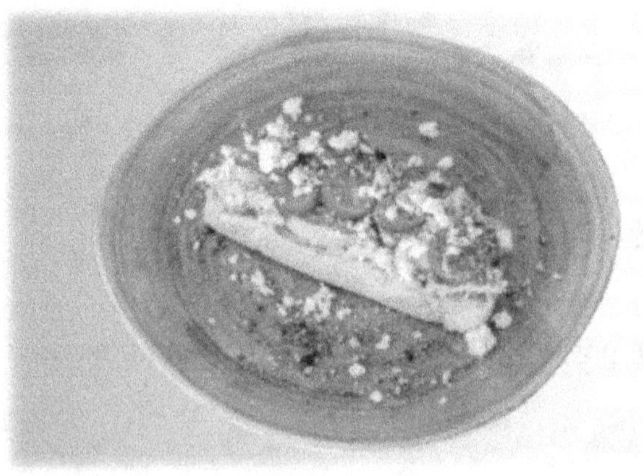

Cottage Cheese and Berry Stuffed Crepes:

<u>Ingredients</u>:

- Whole-grain crepes
- Cottage cheese
- Mixed berries

<u>Instructions</u>:

- Fill the crepes with cottage cheese and berries.
- Serve and enjoy!

<u>Prep Time</u>: 15 minutes

<u>Nutritional Information</u>: Protein-packed and high in antioxidants.

Sweet Potato and Turkey Sausage Skillet:

<u>Ingredients</u>:

- Sweet potatoes
- Lean turkey sausage

- Bell peppers

Instructions:

- Sauté the sweet potatoes, turkey sausage, and peppers until done.
- Serve and enjoy!

Prep Time: 25 minutes

Nutritional Information: Balanced with carbs and lean protein

Blueberry Almond Overnight Oats:

Ingredients:

- Rolled oats
- Unsweetened almond milk
- Blueberries
- Almonds

Instructions:

- Mix the ingredients
- Refrigerate overnight, then garnish with almonds.

Prep Time: 5 minutes (plus overnight soaking)

<u>Nutritional Information</u>: Fiber, antioxidants, and healthy fats

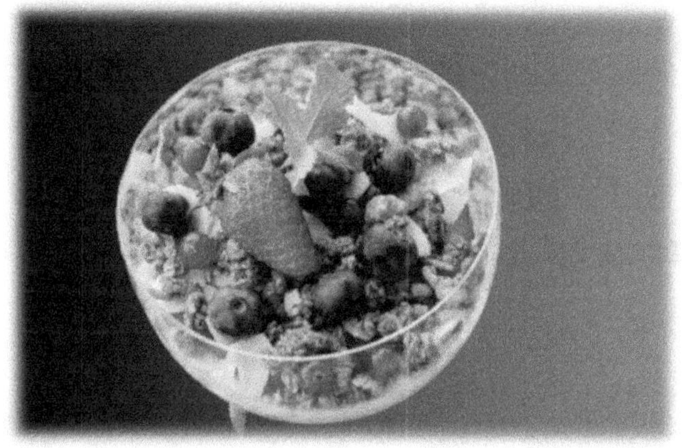

Egg White and Veggie Scramble:

<u>Ingredients</u>:

- Egg whites
- Spinach
- Tomatoes
- Bell peppers

<u>Instructions</u>:

- Sauté the vegetables.

- Add the egg whites then scramble until done.

<u>Prep Time</u>: 10 minutes

<u>Nutritional Information</u>: Low in fat, high in protein

Apple Cinnamon Chia Pudding:

<u>Ingredients</u>:

- Chia seeds
- Unsweetened almond milk
- Apple slices
- Cinnamon

<u>Instructions</u>:

- Mix and allow the chia seeds and almond milk to soak together.
- Top with apple slices and cinnamon.

<u>Prep Time</u>: 10 minutes (plus soaking time)

<u>Nutritional Information</u>: Rich in fiber

Pesto and Tomato Egg Muffins:

<u>Ingredients</u>:

- Eggs

- Cherry tomatoes

- Pesto sauce

Instructions:

- Whisk the eggs.

- Pour into the muffin tin.

- Add the tomatoes and pesto, and bake until done.

Prep Time: 15 minutes

Nutritional Information: Rich in protein

Sausage and Kale Breakfast Casserole:

Ingredients:

- Turkey sausage

- Kale

- Eggs

- Cheese

Instructions:

- Cook the sausage.

- Sauté the kale and stir in eggs.

- Top with cheese and bake.

<u>Prep Time</u>: 30 minutes

<u>Nutritional Information</u>: Balanced with protein and greens

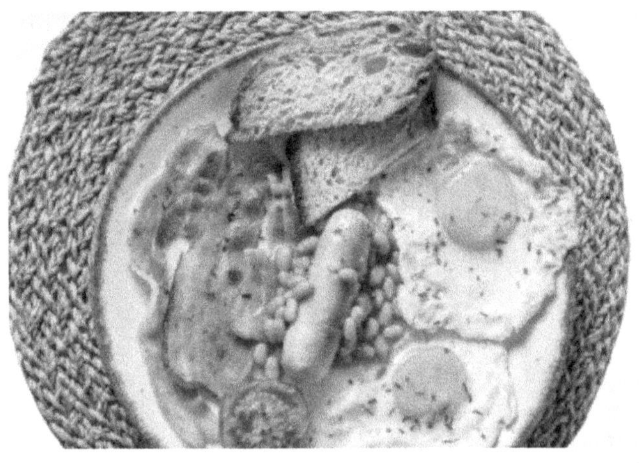

Cranberry Walnut Quinoa Bowl:

<u>Ingredients</u>:

- Cooked quinoa

- Unsweetened cranberries

- Chopped walnuts

<u>Instructions</u>:

- Mix the ingredients.
- Warm if desired, then top with walnuts.

<u>Prep Time</u>: 15 minutes

<u>Nutritional Information</u>: Fiber, antioxidants, and healthy fats

Salmon and Cream Cheese Stuffed Avocado:

<u>Ingredients</u>:

- Smoked salmon
- Cream cheese
- Ripe avocado

<u>Instructions</u>:

- Mix the cream cheese and smoked salmon together.
- Stuff into the halved avocados.

<u>Prep Time</u>: 10 minutes

<u>Nutritional Information</u>: Omega-3 fatty acids and protein

Ricotta and Berry-stuffed French Toast:

<u>Ingredients</u>:

- Whole-grain bread
- Ricotta cheese
- Mixed berries

<u>Instructions</u>:

- Spread the ricotta on the bread.
- Add berries to it, then toast until golden.

<u>Prep Time</u>: 20 minutes

<u>Nutritional Information</u>: Protein and antioxidants

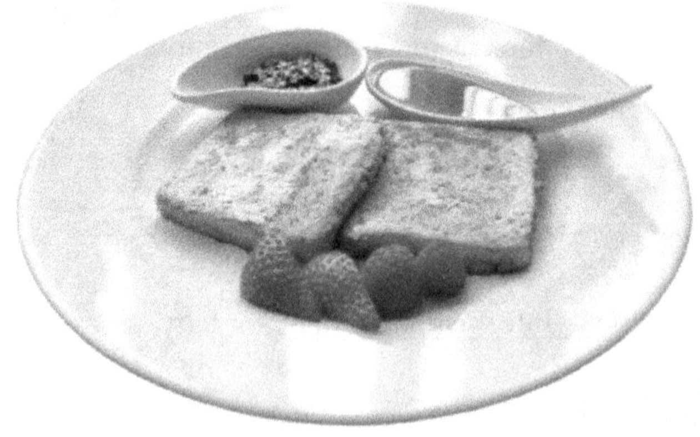

Turmeric and Veggie Scramble:

Ingredients:

- Eggs
- Turmeric
- Bell peppers
- Onions
- Spinach

Instructions:

- Sauté the vegetables.
- Add the eggs and turmeric, and scramble until done.

Prep Time: 15 minutes

Nutritional Information: Vitamins

Chocolate Protein Smoothie:

Ingredients:

- Unsweetened almond milk
- Protein powder
- Chia seeds
- Cocoa powder

<u>Instructions</u>:

- Blend the ingredients together until smooth.
- Serve and enjoy!

<u>Prep Time</u>: 5 minutes

<u>Nutritional Information</u>: High in protein, low in sugar

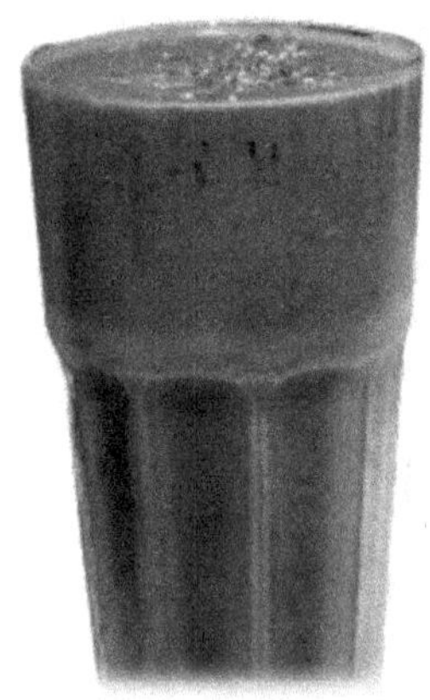

CHAPTER 3: LUNCH RECIPES

Grilled Chicken Salad:

Ingredients:

- Grilled chicken breast
- Mixed salad greens
- Cherry tomatoes
- Cucumber
- Olive oil
- Balsamic vinegar

Instructions:

- Grill the chicken breasts.
- Chop the vegetables and stir them together.
- Drizzle the mixture with olive oil and balsamic vinegar.

Prep Time: 20 minutes

Nutritional Information: Low in carbs, high in protein and fiber

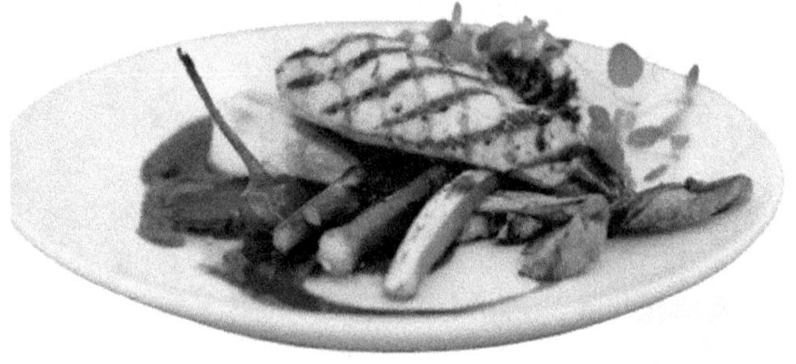

Salmon Quinoa Bowl:

<u>Ingredients</u>:

- Grilled salmon
- Quinoa
- Spinach
- Bell peppers
- Lemon
- Olive oil

<u>Instructions</u>:

- Cook the quinoa.
- Grill the salmon, and sauté the veggies.

- Put it together in a bowl and drizzle with lemon and olive oil.

<u>Prep Time</u>: 25 minutes

<u>Nutritional Information</u>: Rich in omega-3 fatty acids, low in carbs

Vegetable Stir-Fry with Tofu:

<u>Ingredients</u>:

- Tofu
- Broccoli
- Bell peppers
- Snap peas
- Soy sauce
- Garlic
- Ginger

<u>Instructions</u>:

- Sauté the tofu and vegetables with garlic and ginger.
- Stir in soy sauce and stir-fry until soft.

<u>Prep Time</u>: 15 minutes

: High in protein

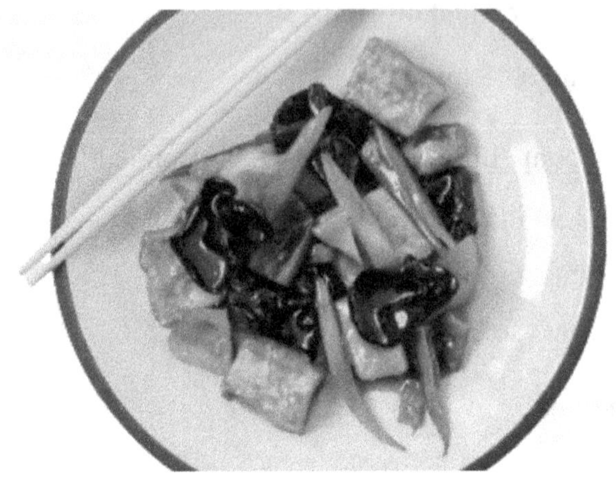

Turkey and Avocado Wrap:

Ingredients:

- Whole grain wrap
- Turkey slices
- Avocado
- Lettuce
- Tomato

Instructions:

- Combine the ingredients in a wrap, roll it up, and cut in half.

Prep Time: 10 minutes

<u>Nutritional Information</u>: Lean protein and healthy fats

Zucchini Noodles with Pesto and Chicken:

<u>Ingredients</u>:

- Zucchini noodles
- Grilled chicken
- Cherry tomatoes
- Homemade pesto

<u>Instructions</u>:

- Spiralize the zucchini.
- Grill the chicken and toss with tomatoes and pesto.

<u>Prep Time</u>: 15 minutes

<u>Nutritional Information</u>: Low in carbs, moderate protein, and healthy fats

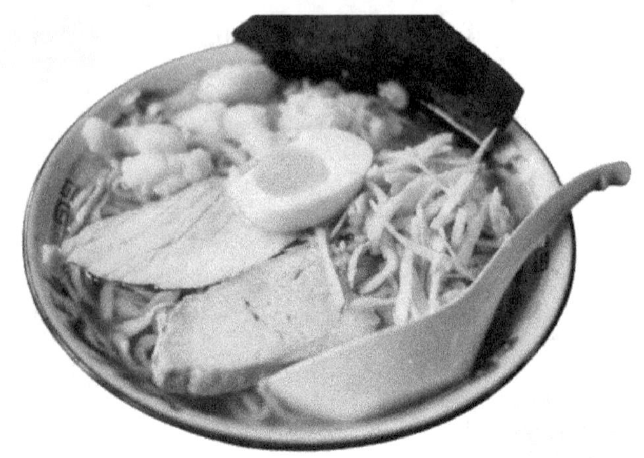

Mediterranean Chickpea Salad:

<u>Ingredients</u>:

- Chickpeas
- Cherry tomatoes
- Cucumber
- Feta cheese
- Olives
- Olive oil
- Lemon juice

<u>Instructions</u>:

- Combine chickpeas and veggies.

- Crumble the feta and drizzle with olive oil and lemon juice.

Prep Time: 15 minutes

Nutritional Information: High in fiber, moderate protein and healthy fats

Egg and Vegetable Stir-Fry:

Ingredients:

- Eggs
- Bell peppers
- Spinach
- Mushrooms
- Onions
- Soy sauce

Instructions:

- Scramble the eggs.
- Stir-fry the vegetables, then add soy sauce until done.

Prep Time: 20 minutes

Nutritional Information: Rich in protein

Quinoa Stuffed Bell Peppers:

Ingredients:

- Quinoa
- Lean ground turkey
- Bell peppers
- Tomatoes
- Spices

Instructions:

- Cook the quinoa and turkey, then stuff the bell peppers and bake them till soft.

Prep Time: 30 minutes

Nutritional Information: Balanced with protein and whole grains

Shrimp and Broccoli Skewers:

Ingredients:

- Shrimp
- Broccoli florets
- Lemon
- Garlic

- Olive oil

<u>Instructions</u>:

- Thread the shrimp and broccoli onto skewers
- Grill them with garlic and lemon.

<u>Prep Time</u>: 15 minutes

<u>Nutritional Information</u>: Low in carbs

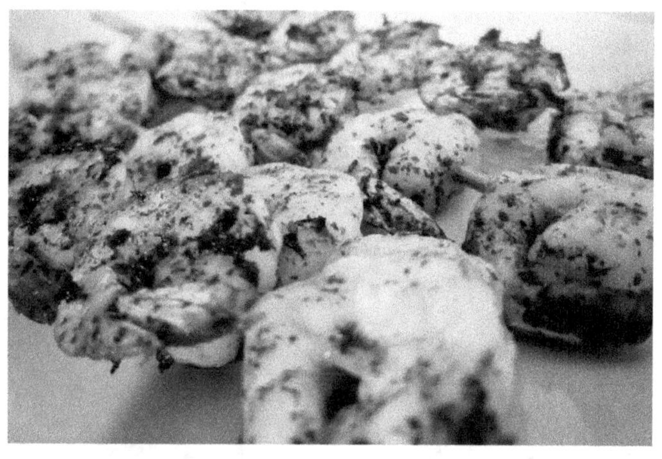

Cauliflower Fried Rice with Chicken:

<u>Ingredients</u>:

- Cauliflower rice
- Chicken breast

- Mixed vegetables

- Soy sauce

<u>Instructions</u>:

- Stir-fry the chicken and vegetables with cauliflower rice and soy sauce.

<u>Prep Time</u>: 25 minutes

<u>Nutritional Information</u>: Low in carbs, high in protein.

Lentil and Vegetable Soup:

<u>Ingredients</u>:

- Lentils

- Carrots

- Celery

- Tomatoes

- Onions

- Low-sodium vegetable broth

<u>Instructions</u>:

- Cook the lentils and vegetables in broth until soft

- Season to taste.

<u>Prep Time</u>: 30 minutes

<u>Nutritional Information</u>: High in fiber

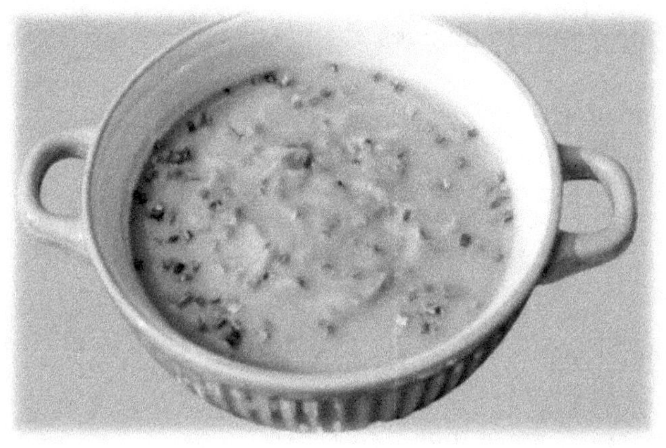

Spinach and Feta Stuffed Chicken Breast:

<u>Ingredients</u>:

- Chicken breast
- Spinach
- Feta cheese
- Garlic
- Herbs

- Butterfly the chicken, then pack it with spinach and feta.
- Bake until thoroughly cooked.

Prep Time: 35 minutes

Nutritional Information: High in protein, low in carbs

Tuna and Avocado Salad:

Ingredients:

- Canned tuna
- Mixed greens
- Cherry tomatoes
- Avocado
- Olive oil

Instructions:

- Combine the tuna, vegetables, and avocado together.
- Drizzle with olive oil.

Prep Time: 15 minutes

<u>Nutritional Information</u>: Rich in omega-3 fatty acids, moderate protein

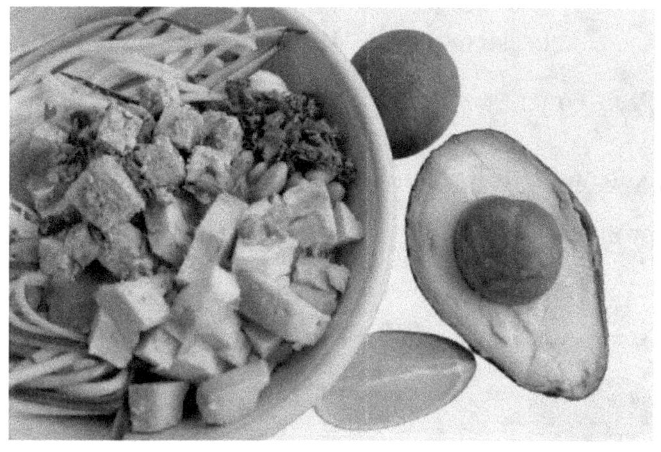

Sweet Potato and Black Bean Quesadilla:

<u>Ingredients</u>:

- Whole grain tortilla
- Sweet potato
- Black beans
- Cheese
- Salsa

<u>Instructions</u>:

- Roast the sweet potatoes and mash them with black beans

- Make the quesadillas and cook until the cheese melts.

<u>Prep Time</u>: 25 minutes

<u>Nutritional Information</u>: High in fiber and moderate protein.

Broccoli and Chicken Alfredo with Brown Rice Pasta:

<u>Ingredients</u>:

- Brown rice pasta
- Chicken breast
- Broccoli
- Homemade Alfredo sauce

<u>Instructions</u>:

- Cook the pasta.

- Sauté the chicken and broccoli, and combine them with the Alfredo sauce.

<u>Prep Time</u>: 30 minutes

Nutritional Information: Balanced with protein and whole grains

Cabbage and Turkey Stir-Fry:

Ingredients:

- Ground turkey
- Cabbage
- Carrots
- Ginger
- Low-sodium soy sauce

Instructions:

- Stir-fry the turkey and vegetables in ginger and soy sauce till done.

Prep Time: 20 minutes

Nutritional Information: High in protein, low in carbs

Caprese Salad with Grilled Chicken:

Ingredients:

- Grilled chicken breast

- Fresh mozzarella

- Tomatoes

- Basil

- Balsamic glaze

<u>Instructions</u>:

- Slice the chicken and layer with mozzarella, tomatoes, and basil.

- Afterwards, drizzle with balsamic glaze.

<u>Prep Time</u>: 15 minutes

<u>Nutritional Information</u>: High in protein, low in carbs

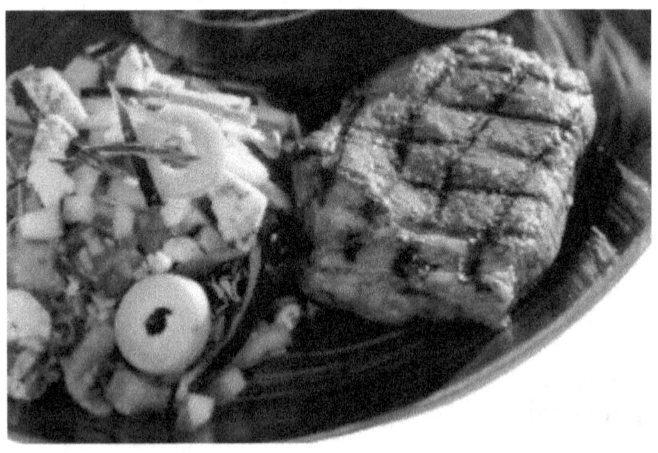

Chickpea and Vegetable Curry:

<u>Ingredients</u>:

- Chickpeas
- Mixed vegetables
- Tomatoes
- Curry spices
- Coconut milk

<u>Instructions</u>:

- Make a curry sauce with tomatoes and coconut milk.
- Cook the chickpeas and vegetables in the curry sauce.

<u>Prep Time</u>: 30 minutes

<u>Nutritional Information</u>: Fiber and protein

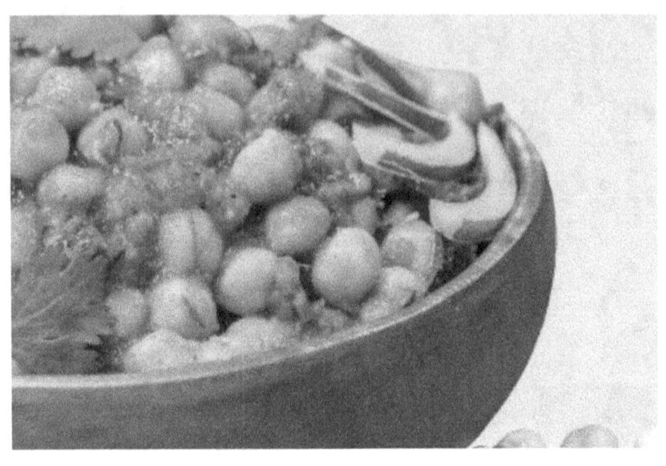

Salmon and Asparagus Foil Packets:

Ingredients:

- Salmon fillets
- Asparagus
- Lemon
- Garlic
- Herbs

Instructions:

- Place the salmon and asparagus on a foil sheet.
- Season with garlic, herbs, and lemon then bake.

<u>Prep Time</u>: 25 minutes

<u>Nutritional Information</u>: Rich in omega-3 fatty acids

Cauliflower and Broccoli Casserole with Chicken:

<u>Ingredients</u>:

- Chicken breast
- Cauliflower
- Broccoli
- Cheese
- Almond flour

<u>Instructions</u>:

- Cook chicken, then mix with steamed cauliflower, broccoli, and cheese.
- Afterwards, bake until golden.

<u>Prep Time</u>: 35 minutes

<u>Nutritional Information</u>: Low in carbs, high in protein

Stuffed Bell Peppers with Turkey and Quinoa:

<u>Ingredients</u>:

- Bell peppers
- Ground turkey
- Quinoa
- Tomatoes
- Spices

<u>Instructions</u>:

- Cook the turkey and quinoa, then mix with the tomatoes and spices.
- Stuff the peppers and bake until soft.

<u>Prep Time</u>: 40 minutes

<u>Nutritional Information</u>: Balanced with protein and whole grains

Shirataki Noodle Stir-Fry with Tofu:

<u>Ingredients</u>:

- Shirataki noodles

- Tofu

- Mixed vegetables

- Soy sauce

- Ginger

Instructions:

- Stir fry the tofu and vegetables with the shirataki noodles.

- Afterwards, add the soy sauce and ginger.

Prep Time: 20 minutes

Nutritional Information: Protein

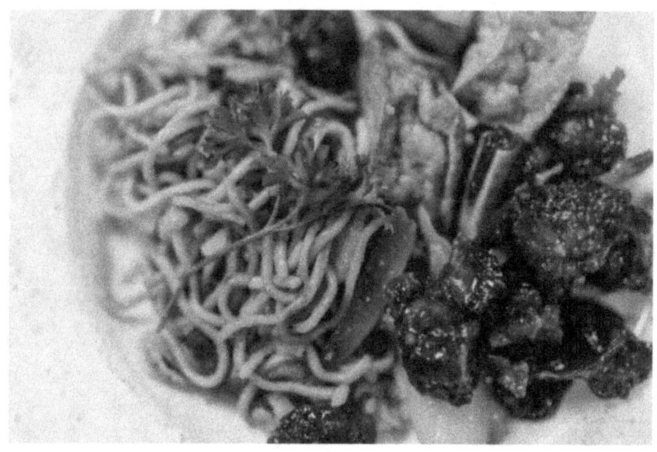

Turkey and Bean Chili:

<u>Ingredients</u>:

- Ground turkey
- Kidney beans
- Tomatoes
- Chili spices
- Onions

<u>Instructions</u>:

- Cook the turkey with onions.
- Afterwards, add the beans, tomatoes, and spices.
- Simmer until the flavors blend.

<u>Prep Time</u>: 30 minutes

<u>Nutritional Information</u>: High in protein and fiber, moderate in carbs

Eggplant and Chickpea Stew:

<u>Ingredients</u>:

- Eggplant
- Chickpeas

- Tomatoes

- Onions

- Garlic

- Cumin

Instructions:

- Sauté the eggplant, onions, and garlic.

- Add the chickpeas, tomatoes, and cumin.

- Simmer until flavors harmonize.

Prep Time: 35 minutes

Nutritional Information: High in fiber

Sesame Ginger Beef Stir-Fry:

Ingredients:

- Lean beef strips

- Broccoli

- Bell peppers

- Snap peas

- Sesame oil

- Ginger

Instructions:

- Stir-fry the beef and vegetables with sesame oil and ginger until done.

<u>Prep Time</u>: 25 minutes

<u>Nutritional Information</u>: High in protein, low in carbs

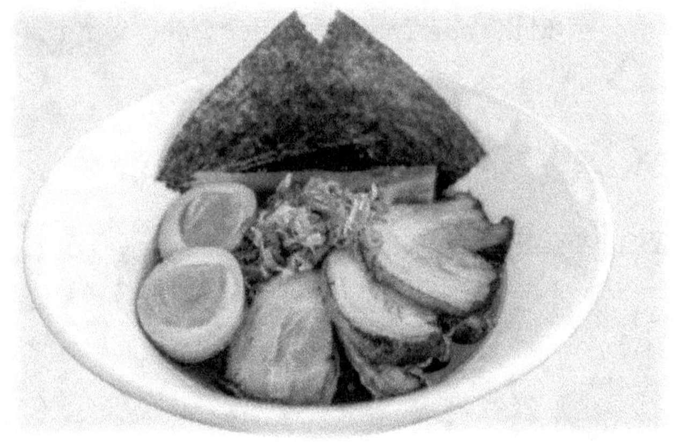

Mushroom and Spinach Frittata:

<u>Ingredients</u>:

- Eggs
- Mushrooms
- Spinach
- Onions

- Feta cheese

<u>Instructions</u>:

- Sauté the vegetables, then pour in the beaten eggs.
- Sprinkle with the feta cheese, and bake until set.

<u>Prep Time</u>: 30 minutes

<u>Nutritional Information</u>: High in protein, low in carbs

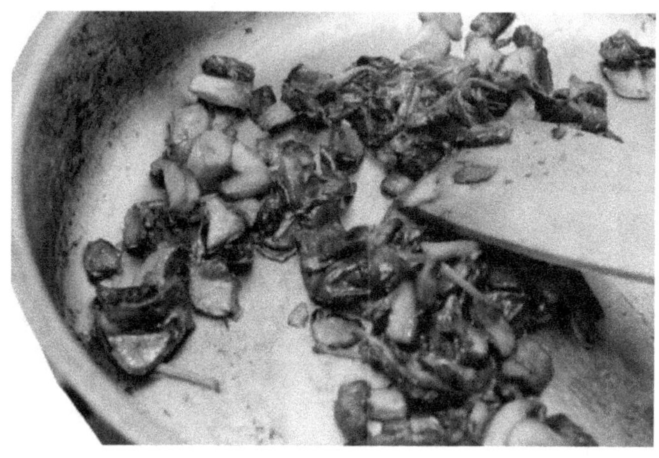

Quinoa and Black Bean Bowl:

<u>Ingredients</u>:

- Quinoa

- Black beans

- Corn

- Avocado

- Lime

- Cilantro

<u>Instructions</u>:

- Cook then quinoa, then mix it with black beans and corn.

- Add avocado, lime, and cilantro as toppings.

<u>Prep Time</u>: 20 minutes

<u>Nutritional Information</u>: Protein and whole grains

CHAPTER 4: DINNER

RECIPES

Grilled Lemon Herb Chicken:

Ingredients:

- Skinless, boneless chicken breasts
- Fresh lemon juice
- Olive oil
- Minced garlic
- Dried oregano
- Salt and pepper

Instructions:

- Make a marinade by mixing lemon juice, olive oil, minced garlic, oregano, salt and pepper together.
- Afterwards, marinate the chicken for 30 minutes.
- Grill till cooked through.

Prep Time: 40 minutes

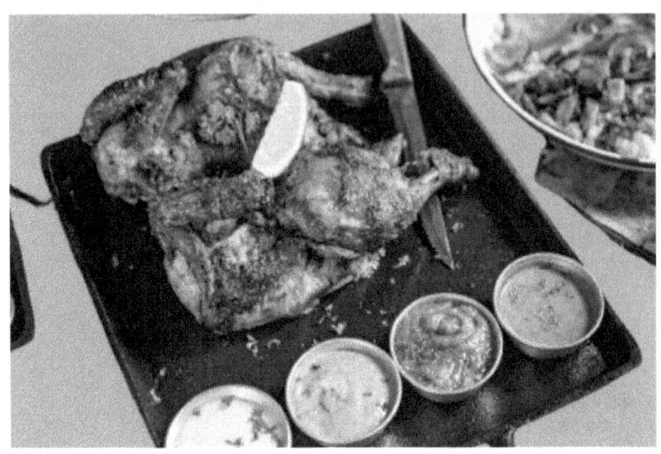

Quinoa and Vegetable Stir-Fry:

Ingredients:

- Quinoa
- Mixed vegetables (bell peppers, broccoli, carrots)
- Low-sodium soy sauce
- Olive oil
- Garlic powder

Instructions:

- Cook the quinoa.

- Stir-fry the vegetables in olive oil with garlic powder.
- Mix in the cooked quinoa and soy sauce.

<u>Prep Time</u>: 25 minutes

<u>Nutritional Information</u>: 300 calories per serving

Baked Salmon with Asparagus:

<u>Ingredients</u>:

- Salmon fillets
- Fresh asparagus
- Lemon slices
- Dijon mustard
- Olive oil
- Minced garlic

<u>Instructions</u>:

- Place the salmon and asparagus on a baking sheet.
- Make a glaze by mixing the Dijon mustard, olive oil, and minced garlic together.
- Bake until the salmon is cooked through.

<u>Prep Time</u>: 30 minutes

<u>Nutritional Information</u>: 280 calories per serving

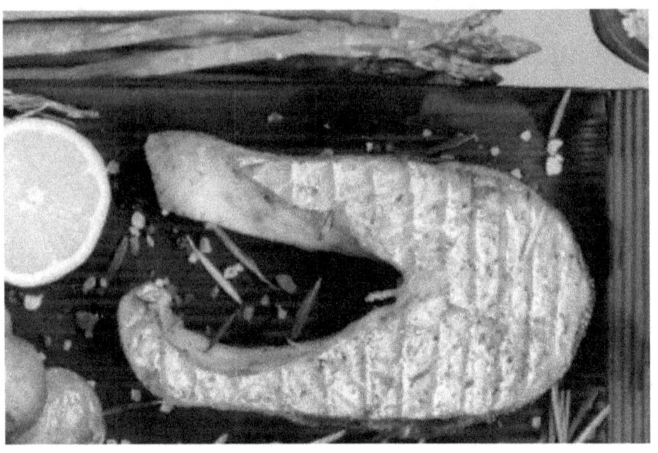

Turkey and Vegetable Skewers:

<u>Ingredients</u>:

- Ground turkey
- Cherry tomatoes
- Zucchini chunks
- Red onion slices
- Olive oil
- Italian seasoning

<u>Instructions</u>:

- Form turkey and veggies on the skewers.

- Brush with olive oil and sprinkle with Italian seasonings.

- Grill the turkey until it is done.

Prep Time: 35 minutes

Nutritional Information: 220 calories per serving

Cauliflower Rice Stir-Fry:

Ingredients:

- Cauliflower rice

- Shrimp or tofu

- Mixed vegetables (broccoli, bell peppers, snap peas)

- Low-sodium teriyaki sauce

- Sesame oil

Instructions:

- Stir-fry the cauliflower rice and vegetables in sesame oil.

- Add the shrimp or tofu, along with the teriyaki sauce.

<u>Prep Time</u>: 20 minutes

<u>Nutritional Information</u>: 230 calories per serving

Chicken and Vegetable Curry:

<u>Ingredients</u>:

- Skinless, boneless chicken thighs
- Mixed vegetables (spinach, bell peppers, cauliflower)
- Coconut milk (light)
- Curry powder
- Turmeric
- Minced ginger

<u>Instructions</u>:

- Sauté the chicken in a pot, then add the vegetables and cook until soft.
- Mix the coconut milk, curry powder, turmeric, and minced ginger.
- Simmer until the flavors merge.

<u>Prep Time</u>: 45 minutes

<u>Nutritional Information</u>: 280 calories per serving

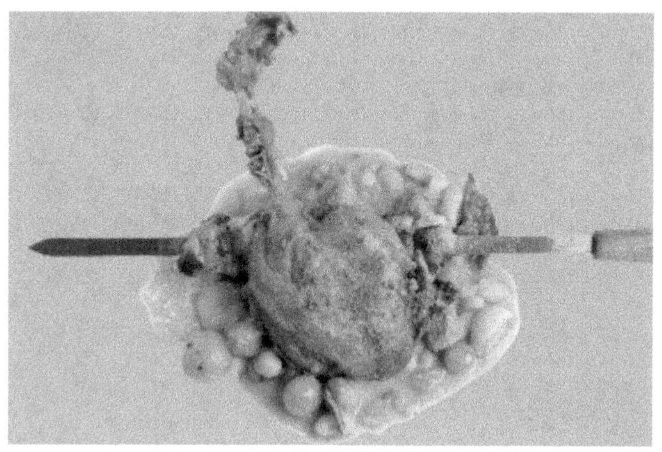

Spinach and Feta Stuffed Chicken:

Ingredients:

- Chicken breasts
- Fresh spinach
- Feta cheese
- Garlic powder
- Lemon zest
- Olive oil

Instructions:

- Butterfly the chicken breasts.
- Stuff it with the spinach, feta, garlic powder, and lemon zest.

- Bake until the chicken is cooked thoroughly.

<u>Prep Time</u>: 35 minutes

<u>Nutritional Information</u>: 260 calories per serving

Zucchini Noodles with Turkey Bolognese:

<u>Ingredients</u>:

- Zucchini noodles
- Ground turkey
- Crushed tomatoes
- Onion, garlic
- Italian seasoning
- Olive oil

<u>Instructions</u>:

- Sauté the turkey, onion, and garlic in olive oil.
- Add crushed tomatoes and Italian seasoning to it.
- Serve with zucchini noodles.

<u>Prep Time</u>: 30 minutes

<u>Nutritional Information</u>: 250 calories per serving

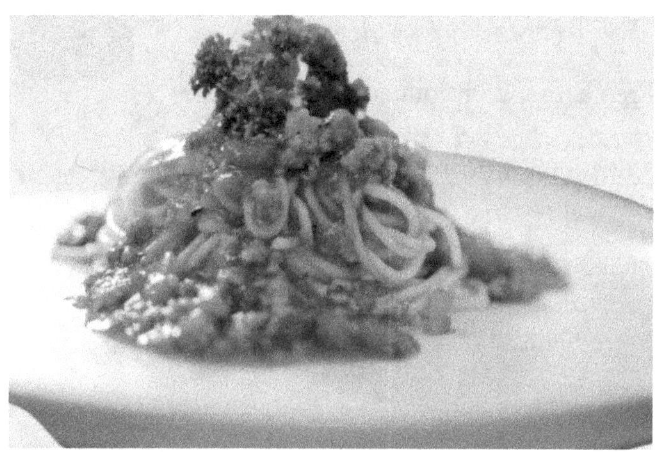

Shrimp and Broccoli Stir-Fry:

<u>Ingredients:</u>

- Shrimp (peeled, deveined)
- Broccoli florets
- Soy sauce (low-sodium)
- Grated ginger
- Minced garlic
- Brown rice

<u>Instructions:</u>

- Stir-fry the shrimp, broccoli, ginger, and garlic.

- Add low-sodium soy sauce and serve with cooked brown rice.

<u>Prep Time</u>: 25 minutes

<u>Nutritional Information</u>: 230 calories per serving

Turkey and Vegetable Lettuce Wraps:

<u>Ingredients</u>:

- Ground turkey

- Lettuce leaves

- Bell peppers, carrots (julienned)

- Hoisin sauce

- Sesame oil

<u>Instructions</u>:

- Cook the ground turkey and add julienned vegetables.

- Mix in the hoisin sauce and sesame oil.

- Then serve with lettuce wraps.

<u>Prep Time</u>: 30 minutes

<u>Nutritional Information</u>: 220 calories per serving

Cauliflower and Chickpea Curry:

<u>Ingredients</u>:

- Cauliflower florets
- Chickpeas (canned, rinsed)
- Coconut milk (light)
- Curry powder
- Turmeric
- Cilantro (chopped)

<u>Instructions</u>:

- Simmer the cauliflower and chickpeas in coconut milk.
- Stir in the curry powder and turmeric.
- Garnish with chopped cilantro.

<u>Prep Time</u>: 40 minutes

<u>Nutritional Information</u>: 250 calories per serving

Greek Chicken Skewers:

<u>Ingredients</u>:

- Chicken breast chunks

- Cherry tomatoes

- Red onion

- Greek seasoning

- Lemon juice

- Olive oil

<u>Instructions</u>:

- Thread the chicken, tomatoes, and onion onto skewers.

- Season with the Greek seasoning, lemon juice, and olive oil.

- Grill the chicken until it is done.

<u>Prep Time</u>: 35 minutes

<u>Nutritional Information</u>: 260 calories per serving

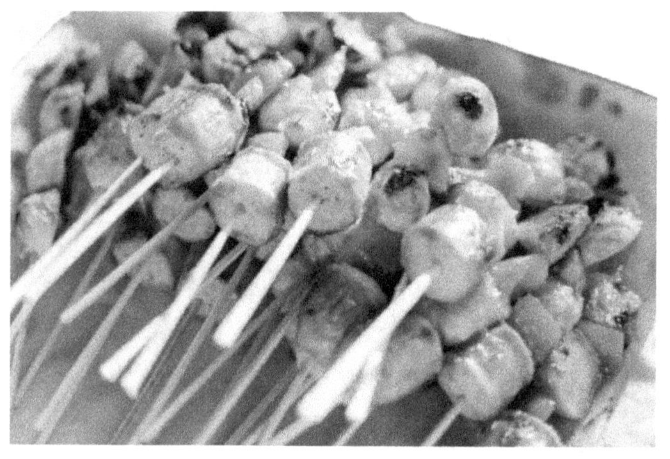

Spinach and Mushroom Stuffed Chicken:

<u>Ingredients:</u>

- Chicken breasts
- Fresh spinach
- Sliced mushrooms
- Minced garlic
- Low-fat mozzarella cheese
- Italian herbs

<u>Instructions:</u>

- Sauté the spinach, mushrooms, and garlic.

- Stuff the chicken breasts with the mixture.

- Bake until the chicken is done, then sprinkle
  with mozzarella and seasonings.

Prep Time: 40 minutes

Nutritional Information: 270 calories per serving

Cabbage and Turkey Sauté:

Ingredients:

- Ground turkey

- Shredded cabbage

- Onion

- Minced garlic

- Low-sodium soy sauce

- Sesame seeds

Instructions:

- Brown the turkey with onions and garlic.

- Combine the shredded cabbage, soy sauce,
  and sesame seeds together.

- Sauté until the cabbage is soft.

Prep Time: 25 minutes

<u>Nutritional Information</u>: 230 calories per serving

Baked Cod with Lemon and Herbs:

<u>Ingredients</u>:

- Cod fillets
- Fresh lemon juice
- Chopped dill
- Garlic powder
- Olive oil

<u>Instructions</u>:

- Place the cod on a baking sheet.
- Drizzle with lemon juice and olive oil, then season with dill and garlic powder.
- Bake until the fish is flaky.

<u>Prep Time</u>: 30 minutes

<u>Nutritional Information</u>: 220 calories per serving

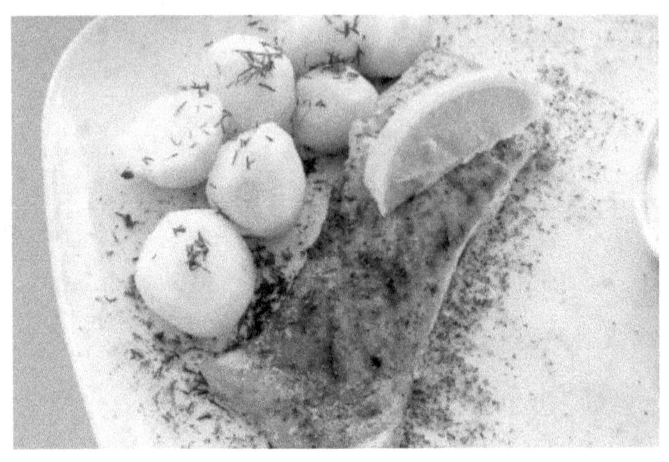

Black Bean and Vegetable Quesadillas:

<u>Ingredients</u>:

- Whole wheat tortillas
- Black beans (canned, rinsed)
- Bell peppers, corn, onions (diced)
- Cumin, chili powder
- Low-fat cheese

<u>Instructions</u>:

- Mix the black beans, diced vegetables, and spices together.

- Spread the mixture on tortillas and top with cheese.

- Cook until the cheese melts.

<u>Prep Time</u>: 25 minutes

<u>Nutritional Information</u>: 260 calories per serving

Spaghetti Squash with Turkey Meatballs:

<u>Ingredients</u>:

- Spaghetti squash

- Ground turkey

- Tomato sauce (no added sugar)

- Italian herbs

- Parmesan cheese (grated)

<u>Instructions</u>:

- Roast the spaghetti squash and shred it into strands.

- Form turkey meatballs, bake, and then boil in tomato sauce.

- Serve over spaghetti squash, topped with herbs and Parmesan.

<u>Prep Time</u>: 45 minutes

<u>Nutritional Information</u>: 290 calories per serving

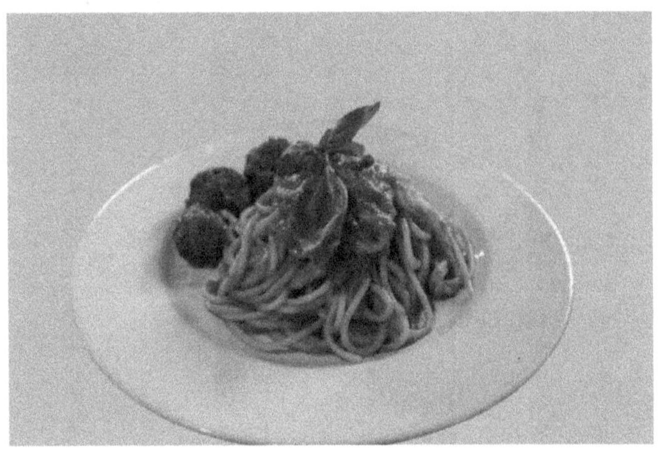

Broccoli and Chicken Skillet:

<u>Ingredients</u>:

- Chicken thighs (skinless, boneless)
- Broccoli florets
- Lemon zest
- Chicken broth (low-sodium)
- Garlic (minced)

- Olive oil

Instructions:

- Sauté the chicken in olive oil until browned.
- Mix broccoli, garlic, lemon zest, and chicken broth together.
- Simmer until the chicken is done and the broccoli is soft.

Prep Time: 30 minutes

Nutritional Information: 250 calories per serving

Veggie and Turkey Stuffed Pepper:

Ingredients:

- Ground turkey
- Bell peppers
- Quinoa
- Tomatoes (diced)
- Cumin, paprika
- Low-fat cheddar cheese

Instructions:

- Cook the turkey, quinoa, tomatoes, and spices.

- Stuff bell peppers with the mixture and top with cheese.

- Bake until the peppers are soft.

Prep Time: 40 minutes

Nutritional Information: 270 calories per serving

Lemon Garlic Shrimp with Zoodles:

Ingredients:

- Shrimp (peeled, deveined)

- Zucchini noodles

- Lemon juice

- Garlic (minced)

- Fresh parsley

- Olive oil

Instructions:

- Sauté the shrimp in olive oil with garlic.

- Combine the noodles, lemon juice, and parsley.

- Cook until the prawns are pink and the noodles are soft.

<u>Prep Time</u>: 25 minutes

<u>Nutritional Information</u>: 240 calories per serving

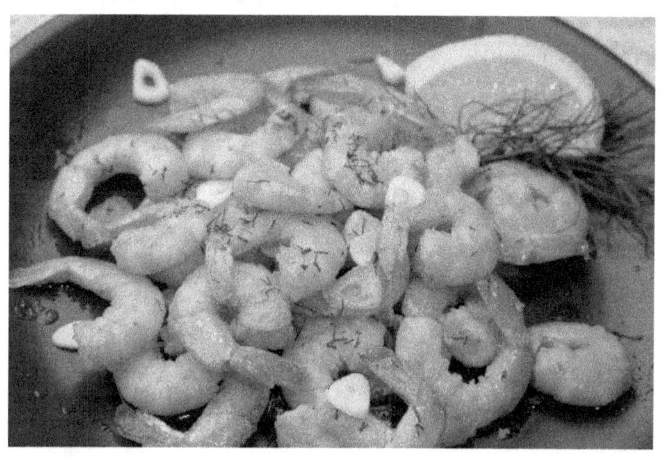

Turkey and Sweet Potato Hash:

<u>Ingredients</u>:

- Ground turkey

- Sweet potatoes (diced)

- Bell peppers, onions (diced)

- Smoked paprika, cumin

- Olive oil

Instructions:

- Brown the turkey in olive oil, then add the cubed sweet potatoes, peppers, and onion.
- Season with smoked paprika and cumin.
- Cook until the sweet potatoes are soft.

Prep Time: 35 minutes

Nutritional Information: 230 calories per serving

Grilled Veggie and Chicken Kabobs:

Ingredients:

- Chicken breast chunks
- Bell peppers, cherry tomatoes, zucchini
- Balsamic vinegar
- Italian seasoning
- Olive oil

Instructions:

- Thread the chicken and vegetables onto the skewers.
- Combine balsamic vinegar, Italian spice, and olive oil together.

- Grill until the chicken is done and the vegetables are soft.

Prep Time: 30 minutes

Nutritional Information: 260 calories per serving

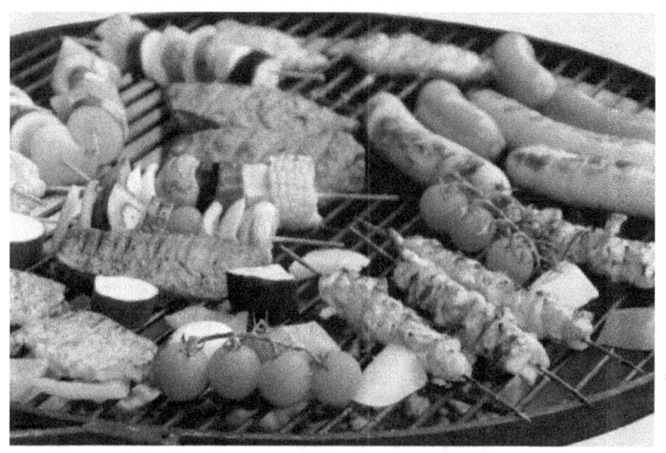

Sesame Ginger Tofu Stir-Fry:

Ingredients:

- Extra-firm tofu (cubed)

- Broccoli florets

- Snap peas

- Low-sodium soy sauce

- Sesame oil

- Fresh ginger (grated)

<u>Instructions</u>:

- Sauté the tofu till golden, then add vegetables.
- Mix soy sauce, sesame oil, and grated ginger together.
- Stir-fry until the vegetables are crisp-tender.

<u>Prep Time</u>: 30 minutes

<u>Nutritional Information</u>: 220 calories per serving

CHAPTER 5: SNACKS AND DESSERT RECIPES

Almond and Berry Yogurt Parfait:

Ingredients:

- Greek yogurt
- Almonds
- Mixed berries
- Honey

Instructions:

- Layer the yogurt, berries, and almonds.
- Drizzle with honey and repeat the process.

Prep Time: 5 minutes

Nutritional Information: Low sugar and high in fiber

Cucumber and Hummus Bites:

Ingredients:

- Cucumber slices

- Hummus

Instructions:

- Spread the hummus on the cucumber slices, then serve.

Prep Time: 10 minutes

Nutritional Information: Low carb, high in fiber, moderate protein

Avocado Chocolate Mousse:

Ingredients:

- Avocado
- Cocoa powder
- Almond milk
- Vanilla extract

Instructions:

- Blend the ingredients together until you get a smooth texture.

Prep Time: 15 minutes

Nutritional Information: Healthy fats, low sugar

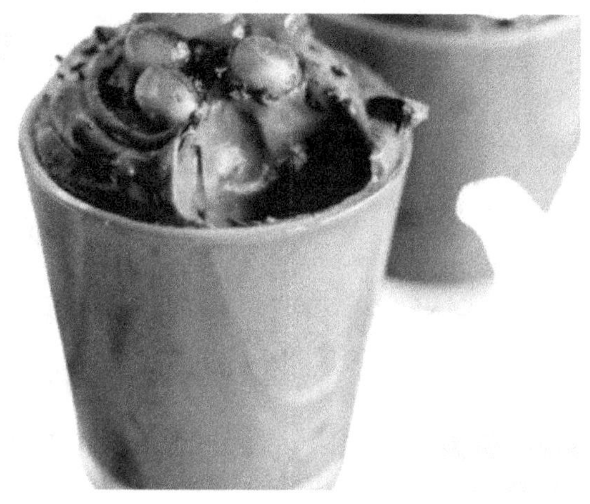

Baked Sweet Potato Chips:

<u>Ingredients</u>:

- Sweet potatoes
- Olive oil
- Sea salt

<u>Instructions</u>:

- Slice the sweet potatoes, toss them with oil
- Afterwards, bake them until crispy.

<u>Prep Time</u>: 20 minutes

<u>Nutritional Information</u>: Moderate carbs

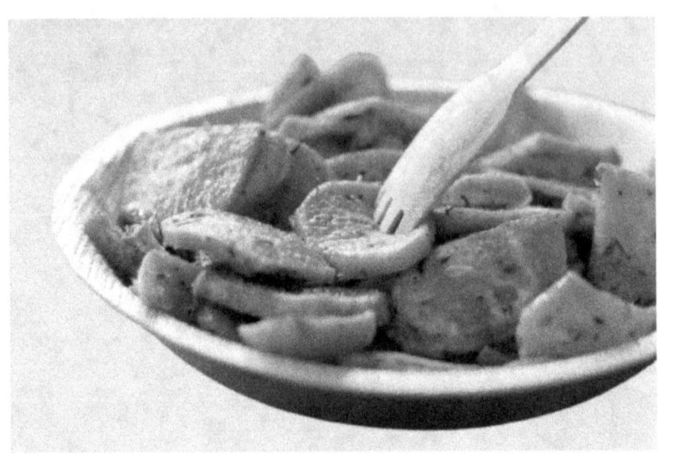

Spinach and Feta Stuffed: Mushrooms:

<u>Ingredients</u>:

- Mushrooms
- Spinach
- Feta cheese
- Garlic

<u>Instructions</u>:

- Sauté the spinach and garlic, then pack the mushrooms and bake.

<u>Prep Time</u>: 25 minutes

<u>Nutritional Information</u>: Low in carb, high in fiber

89

Strawberry and Spinach Salad:

<u>Ingredients</u>:

- Spinach
- Strawberries
- Feta cheese
- Balsamic vinaigrette

<u>Instructions</u>:

- Toss the ingredients together, then drizzle with vinaigrette.

<u>Prep Time</u>: 10 minutes

<u>Nutritional Information</u>: Low in carb, high in fiber

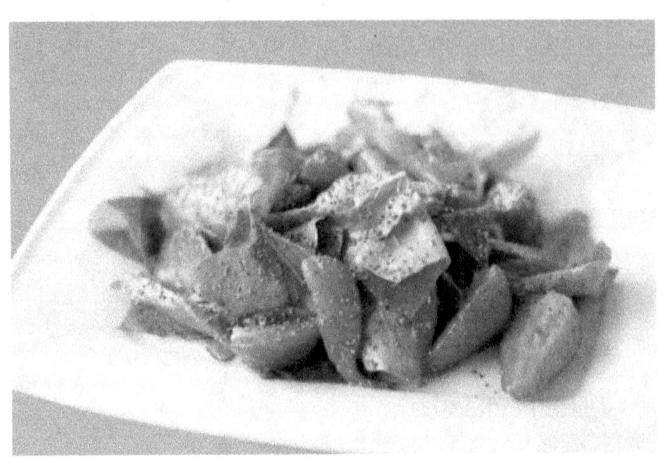

Quinoa and Black Bean Stuffed Peppers:

Ingredients:

- Quinoa
- Black beans
- Bell peppers
- Salsa

Instructions:

- Cook the quinoa, then mix with beans and salsa.
- Stuff the peppers.

<u>Prep Time</u>: 30 minutes

<u>Nutritional Information</u>: High in fiber, moderate protein

Cauliflower Pizza Bites:

<u>Ingredients</u>:

- Cauliflower
- Eggs
- Cheese
- Tomato sauce

<u>Instructions</u>:

- Make a cauliflower crust.
- Top it with sauce and cheese, then bake.

<u>Prep Time</u>: 35 minutes

<u>Nutritional Information</u>: Moderate protein

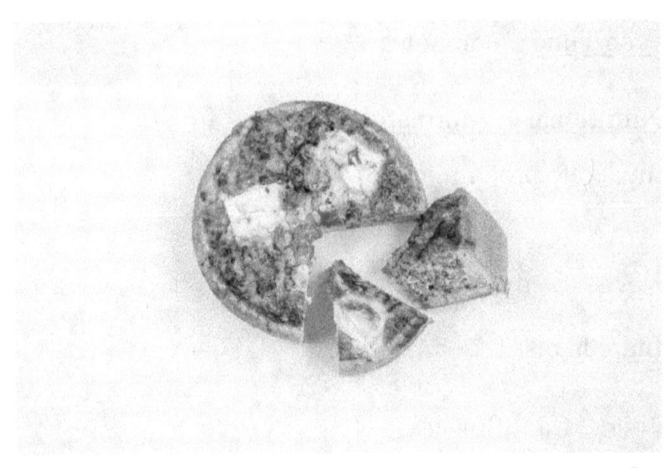

Lemon Blueberry Oat Bars:

Ingredients:

- Oats
- Almond flour
- Blueberries
- Lemon zest

Instructions:

- Mix the ingredients together.
- Flatten into bars, then bake.

Prep Time: 25 minutes

Nutritional Information: High in fiber, low sugar

Sliced Apple with Peanut Butter:

Ingredients:

- Apple slices
- Natural peanut butter

Instructions:

- Spread peanut butter over apple slices, then serve.

Prep Time: 5 minutes

Nutritional Information: Healthy fats

Tuna Salad Lettuce Wraps:

Ingredients:

- Tuna
- Mayonnaise
- Celery
- Lettuce leaves

Instructions:

- Mix the tuna, mayonnaise, and celery together

- Spread onto lettuce leaves and serve.

<u>Prep Time</u>: 15 minutes

<u>Nutritional Information</u>: High protein, low carb

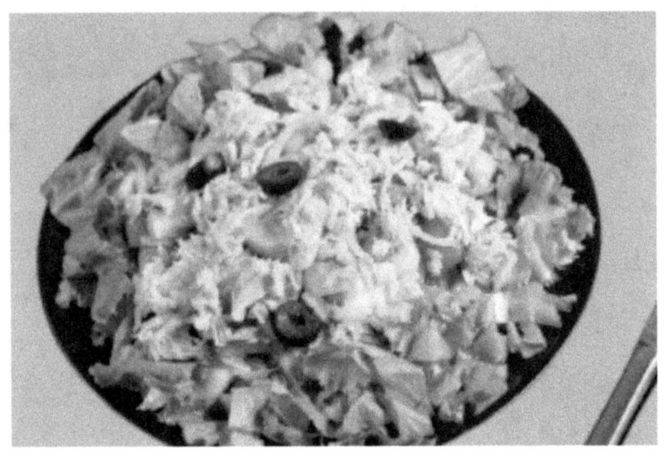

Greek Yogurt with Nuts and Berries:

<u>Ingredients</u>:

- Greek yogurt
- Mixed nuts
- Berries

<u>Instructions</u>:

- Top the yogurt with nuts and berries, then serve.

<u>Prep Time</u>: 5 minutes

<u>Nutritional Information</u>: High in protein and low sugar

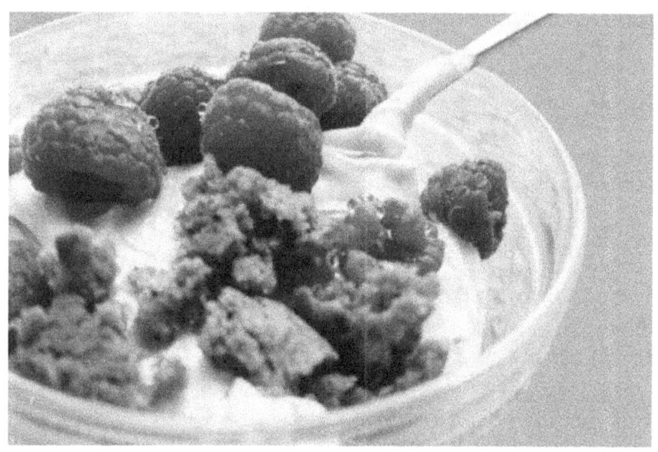

Roasted Chickpeas:

<u>Ingredients</u>:

- Chickpeas
- Olive oil
- Spices

<u>Instructions</u>:

- Toss the chickpeas with oil and spices, then roast until crispy.

Prep Time: 40 minutes

Nutritional Information: High fiber and moderate protein

Baked Zucchini Chips:

Ingredients:

- Zucchini
- Parmesan cheese
- Olive oil

Instructions:

- Slice the zucchini and coat with oil and cheese
- Afterwards, bake it.

Prep Time: 30 minutes

Nutritional Information: Low carb, moderate protein

Salmon and Cucumber Roll-Ups:

Ingredients:

- Smoked salmon

- Cucumber

- Cream cheese

<u>Instructions</u>:

- Spread the cream cheese on the cucumber slices and roll with salmon.

<u>Prep Time</u>: 10 minutes

<u>Nutritional Information</u>: Protein and healthy fats

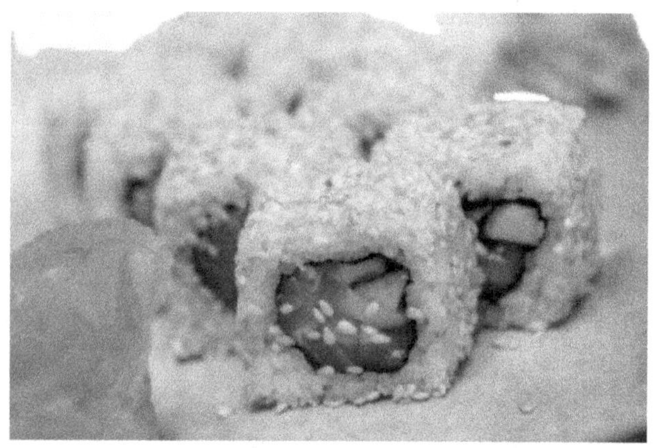

Mango and Chili Lime Shrimp Skewers:

<u>Ingredients</u>:

- Shrimp

- Mango

- Lime juice

- Chili powder

Instructions:

- Set the shrimp and mango onto the skewer.

- Afterwards, grill them with lime and chili.

Prep Time: 20 minutes

Nutritional Information: High protein, low sugar

Walnut and Berry Salad:

Ingredients:

- Mixed greens

- Walnuts

- Mixed berries

- Vinaigrette

Instructions:

- Toss the greens, berries, and walnuts.

- Drizzle with vinaigrette afterwards.

Prep Time: 15 minutes

<u>Nutritional Information</u>: Healthy fats

Broccoli and Cheese Bites:

<u>Ingredients</u>:

- Broccoli
- Cheddar cheese
- Eggs

<u>Instructions</u>:

- Mix the ingredients together and shape it into bits then bake.

<u>Prep Time</u>: 25 minutes

<u>Nutritional Information</u>: High fiber, moderate protein

Peanut Butter Banana Smoothie:

<u>Ingredients</u>:

- Banana
- Peanut butter
- Almond milk
- Ice

<u>Instructions</u>:

- Blend the ingredients together until you get a smooth feel.

<u>Prep Time</u>: 5 minutes

<u>Nutritional Information</u>: Moderate carbs, healthy fats

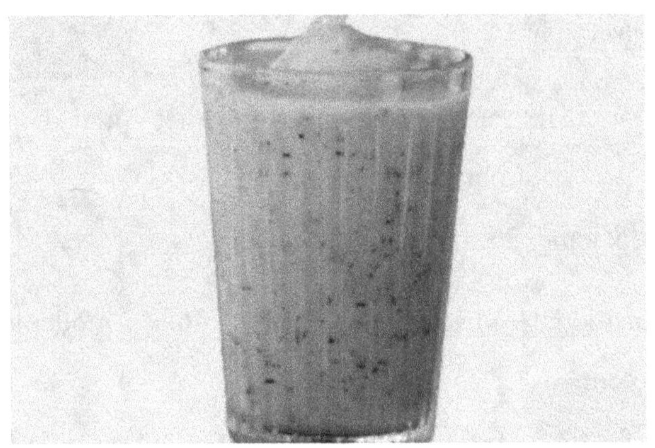

Eggplant and Tomato Stacks:

<u>Ingredients</u>:

- Eggplant
- Tomatoes
- Mozzarella cheese

- Basil

<u>Instructions</u>:

- Layer the eggplant, tomatoes, and cheese in a baking pan then bake.

<u>Prep Time</u>: 30 minutes

<u>Nutritional Information</u>: Low carb, moderate protein

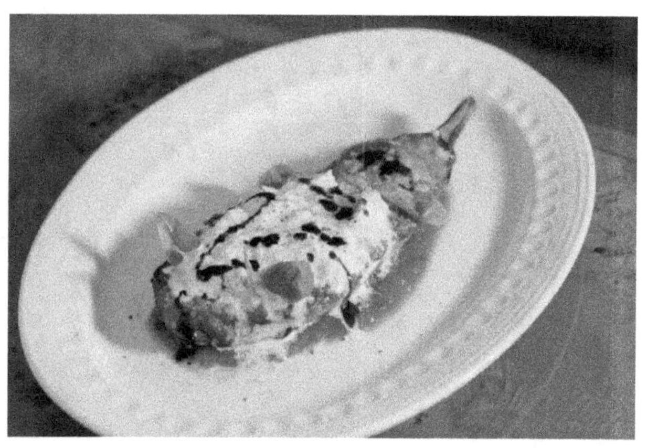

Cherry Almond Energy Balls:

<u>Ingredients</u>:

- Dates

- Almonds

- Dried cherries

Instructions:

- Mix and blend the ingredients then shape into balls.

Prep Time: 15 minutes

Nutritional Information: High fiber and low sugar

Mushroom and Spinach Omelet:

Ingredients:

- Egg
- Mushrooms
- Spinach
- Feta cheese

Instructions:

- Cook the mushrooms and spinach, then add the beaten eggs and simmer.

Prep Time: 15 minutes

Nutritional Information: High protein, low carb

Brussels Sprouts and Bacon Skewers:

Ingredients:

- Brussels sprouts
- Bacon
- Olive oil

Instructions:

- Wrap the sprouts with bacon
- Afterwards skewer them and cook.

Prep Time: 20 minutes

Nutritional Information: Low carb, moderate protein

Lemon Garlic Roasted Asparagus:

Ingredients:

- Asparagus
- Lemon
- Garlic
- Olive oil

Instructions:

- Toss the asparagus with oil, lemon, and garlic, then roast.

Prep Time: 15 minutes

Nutritional Information: Low carb and high fiber

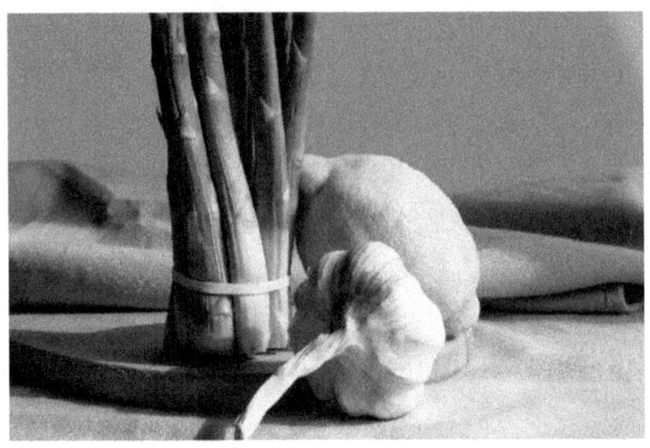

Cottage Cheese and Pineapple Bowl:

Ingredients:

- Cottage cheese
- Pineapple chunks

Instructions:

- Mix the cottage cheese with the pineapple chunks, then serve.

<u>Prep Time</u>: 5 minutes

<u>Nutritional Information</u>: High protein and moderate carbs

Dark Chocolate-Dipped Strawberries:

<u>Ingredients</u>:

- Dark chocolate
- Strawberries

<u>Instructions</u>:

- Melt the chocolate.
- Immerse the strawberries in the chocolate and let them set.

<u>Prep Time</u>: 15 minute

<u>Nutritional Information</u>: Antioxidants

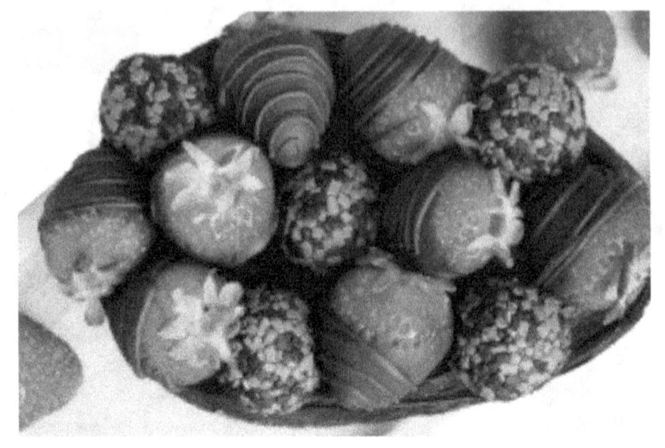

Mango Salsa with Baked Pita Chips:

Ingredients:

- Mango
- Tomatoes
- Red onion
- Whole wheat pita

Instructions:

- Dice the ingredients and make the salsa.
- Afterwards, bake the pita chips.

Prep Time: 25 minutes

Nutritional Information: High fiber

CHAPTER 6: SMOOTHIE RECIPES

Mango Tango Smoothie:

Ingredients:

- Mango chunks
- Plain yogurt
- Hemp seeds
- Turmeric
- Water

Instructions:

- Blend all the ingredients together until creamy.
- Serve and enjoy!

Prep Time: 6 minutes

Nutritional Information: Carbs, fiber, calories and protein

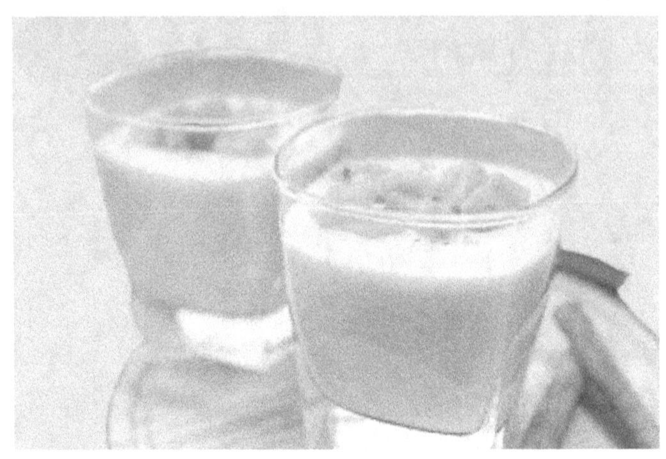

Cinnamon Apple Delight:

Ingredients:

- Apple (peeled and sliced)
- Cinnamon
- Almond butter
- Unsweetened soy milk

Instructions:

- Blend all the ingredients together until you get a smooth feel.
- Serve and enjoy!

Prep Time: 5 minutes

<u>Nutritional Information</u>: Carbs, fiber, calories and protein

Cherry Almond Bliss:

<u>Ingredients</u>:

- Cherries
- Almonds
- Cottage cheese
- Flaxseed oil
- Unsweetened almond milk

<u>Instructions</u>:

- Blend all the ingredients together until you get a smooth feel.
- Serve and enjoy!

<u>Prep Time</u>: 8 minutes

<u>Nutritional Information</u>: Carbs, fiber, calories and protein

Green Power Smoothie:

<u>Ingredients</u>:

- Spinach
- Avocado
- Cucumber
- Parsley
- Flaxseeds
- Coconut water

<u>Instructions:</u>

- Blend all the ingredients together until creamy.
- Serve and enjoy!

<u>Prep Time:</u> 7 minutes

<u>Nutritional Information:</u> Carbs, fiber and protein

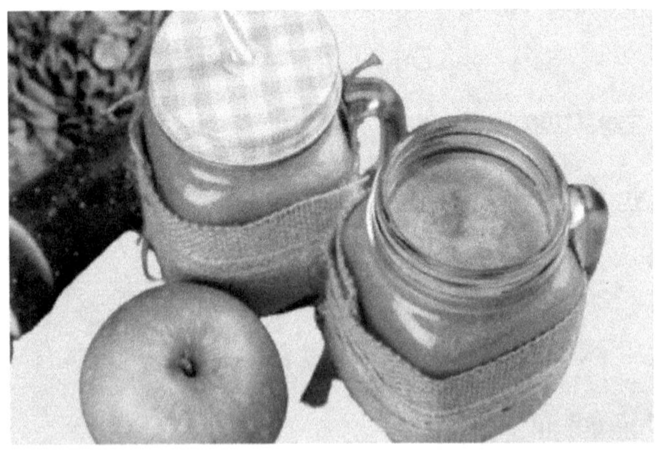

Blueberry Basil Bliss:

<u>Ingredients</u>:

- Blueberries
- Fresh basil leaves
- Plain yogurt
- Flaxseeds
- Water

<u>Instructions</u>:

- Blend all the ingredients together until you get a smooth feel.
- Serve and enjoy!

<u>Prep Time</u>: 6 minutes

<u>Nutritional Information</u>: Carbs, fiber, calories and protein

Berry Bliss Smoothie:

<u>Ingredients</u>:

- Mixed berries (strawberries, blueberries, raspberries)
- Banana

- Greek yogurt

- Chia seeds

- Unsweetened almond milk

Instructions:

- Blend all the ingredients together until you get a smooth feel.

- Serve and enjoy!

Prep Time: 5 minutes

Nutritional Information: Calories, carbs, fiber and protein

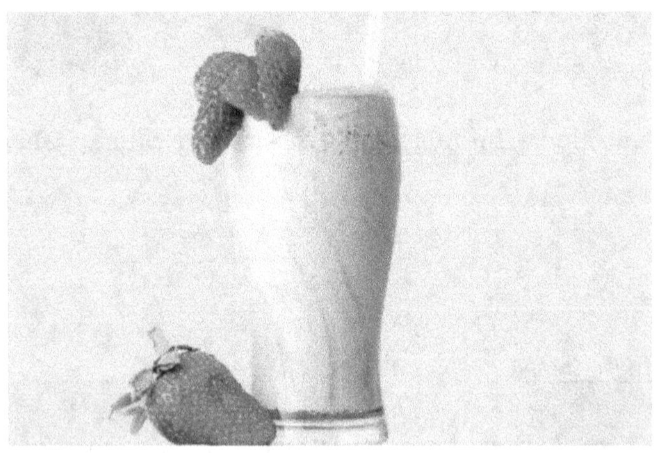

Avocado Lime Zest:

<u>Ingredients</u>:

- Avocado
- Lime juice
- Chia seeds
- Spinach
- Unsweetened soy milk

<u>Instructions</u>:

- Blend all the ingredients together until creamy.
- Serve and enjoy!

<u>Prep Time</u>: 5 minutes

<u>Nutritional Information</u>: Carbs, fiber, calories and protein

Vanilla Almond Dream:

<u>Ingredients</u>:

- Vanilla extract
- Almonds
- Greek yogurt

- Almond butter
- Unsweetened almond milk

Instructions:

- Blend all the ingredients together until you get a smooth feel.
- Serve and enjoy!

Prep Time: 7 minutes

Nutritional Information: Carbs, fiber, calories and protein

Peachy Keen Smoothie:

Ingredients:

- Sliced peaches
- Plain yogurt
- Chia seeds
- Ginger
- Unsweetened soy milk

Instructions:

- Blend all the ingredients together until you get a smooth feel.

- Serve and enjoy!

<u>Prep Time</u>: 6 minutes

<u>Nutritional Information</u>: Carbs, fiber, calories and protein

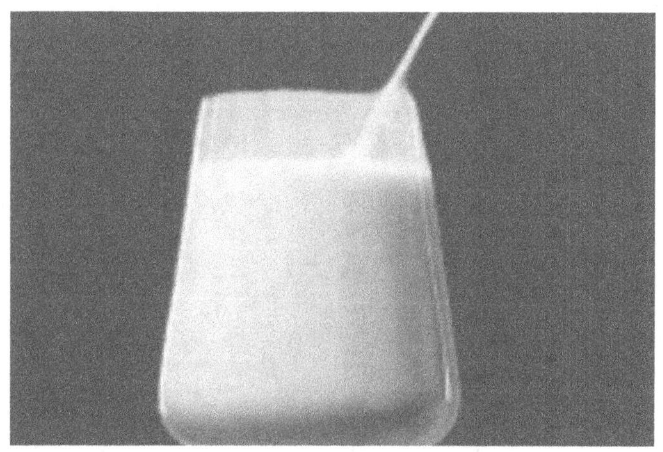

Raspberry Coconut Refresher:

<u>Ingredients</u>:

- Raspberries
- Coconut milk
- Hemp seeds
- Banana
- Water

<u>Instructions</u>:

- Blend all of the ingredients together until it is creamy.
- Serve and enjoy!

<u>Prep Time</u>: 7 minutes

<u>Nutritional Information</u>: Carbs, fiber, calories and protein

Carrot Cake Smoothie:

<u>Ingredients</u>:

- Shredded carrots
- Cinnamon
- Almond butter
- Banana
- Unsweetened almond milk

<u>Instructions</u>:

- Blend all of the ingredients together until you get a smooth feel.
- Serve and enjoy!

<u>Prep Time</u>: 6 minutes

<u>Nutritional Information</u>: Carbs, fiber, calories and protein

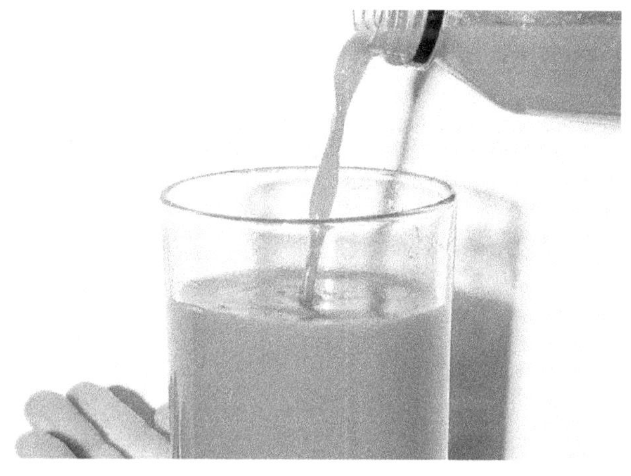

Coconut Mint Cooler:

<u>Ingredients</u>:

- Coconut water
- Mint leaves
- Almonds
- Banana
- Coconut milk

<u>Instructions</u>:

- Blend all of the ingredients together until it
  is creamy.
- Serve and enjoy!

<u>Prep Time</u>: 6 minutes

<u>Nutritional Information</u>: Calories, carbs and protein

CHAPTER 7: SALAD RECIPES

Grilled Chicken and Avocado Salad:

Ingredients:

- Grilled chicken breast
- Mixed greens
- Cherry tomatoes
- Cucumber
- Avocado

Instructions:

- Grill the chicken and cut the vegetables.
- Blend them together and serve with sliced avocado.

Prep Time: 20 minutes

Nutritional Information: High in protein and fiber

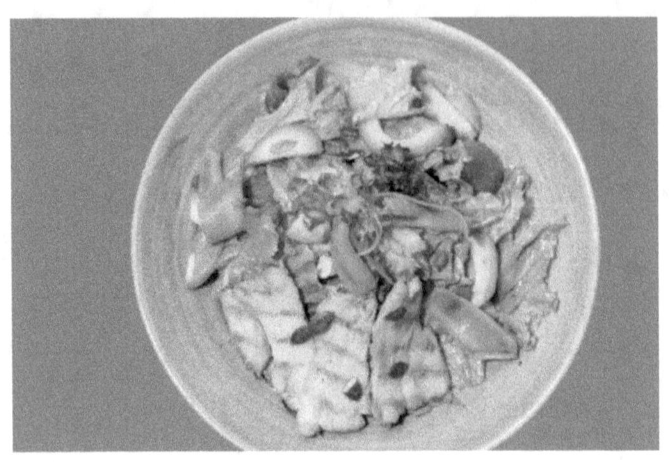

Roasted Vegetable Salad:

Ingredients:

- Assorted veggies (zucchini, bell peppers, cherry tomatoes)
- Mixed greens
- Balsamic glaze

Instructions:

- Roast the vegetables and toss in the greens.
- Drizzle the mix with balsamic glaze.

Prep Time: 30 minutes

<u>Nutritional Information</u>: Low in carbs, high in vitamins

Salmon and Spinach Salad:

<u>Ingredients</u>:

- Baked salmon
- Baby spinach
- Red bell pepper
- Feta cheese
- Olive oil

<u>Instructions</u>:

- Bake the salmon and mix it with spinach.
- Add the chopped pepper to it, sprinkle the mix with the feta cheese, then drizzle with oil.

<u>Prep Time</u>: 25 minutes

<u>Nutritional Information</u>: Rich in omega-3

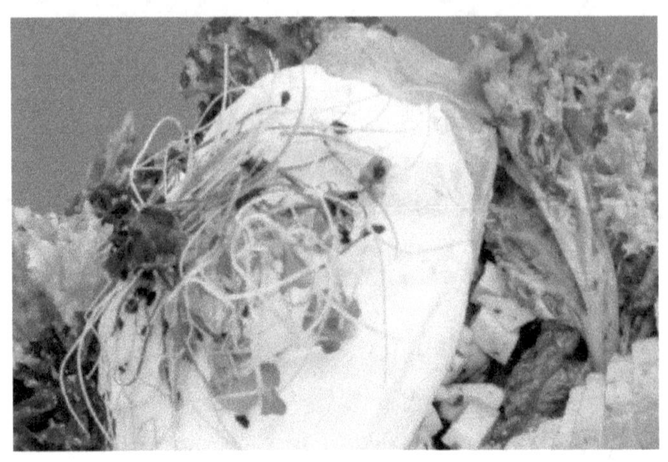

Mediterranean Quinoa Salad:

<u>Ingredients:</u>

- Quinoa

- Cherry tomatoes

- Cucumbers

- Olives

- Feta

- Olive oil

<u>Instructions:</u>

- Cook the quinoa, then mix it with the chopped veggies.

- Add olives and feta to the mix then finish it off by drizzling with olive oil.

Prep Time: 30 minutes

Nutritional Information: High in fiber and moderate in carbs

Shrimp and Asparagus Salad:

Ingredients:

- Grilled shrimp
- Asparagus
- Mixed greens
- Cherry tomatoes
- Lemon vinaigrette

Instructions:

- Grill the shrimp and asparagus, then mix with the greens.
- Add the tomatoes and dress with lemon vinaigrette.

Prep Time: 20 minutes

Nutritional Information: High in protein

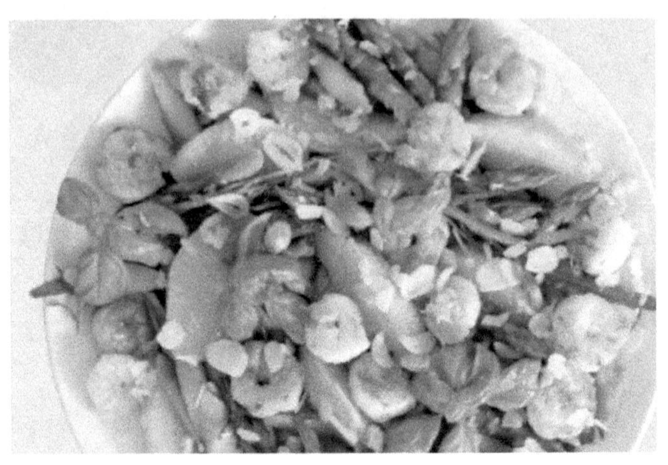

Cauliflower and Broccoli Salad:

<u>Ingredients</u>:

- Steamed cauliflower and broccoli
- Red onion
- Feta
- Greek yogurt dressing

<u>Instructions</u>:

- Steam the vegetables, then mix with the red onion and feta before tossing in the Greek yogurt dressing.

<u>Prep Time</u>: 15 minutes

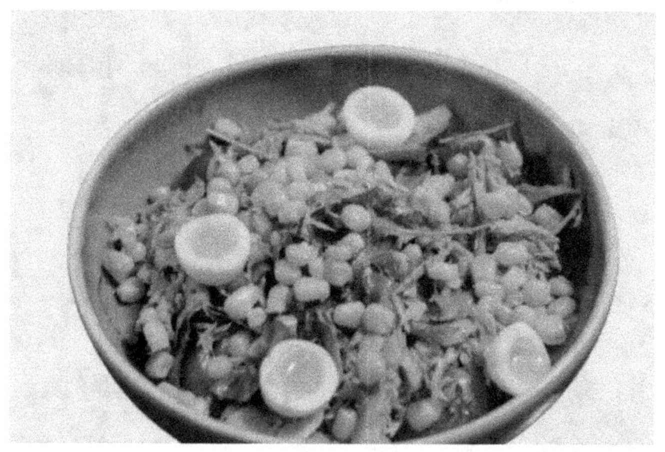

Greek Salad with Chicken:

Ingredients:

- Grilled chicken
- Romaine lettuce
- Cherry tomatoes
- Olives, feta
- Greek dressing

Instructions:

- Grill the chicken, then toss it with lettuce, tomatoes, olives, and feta.

- Drizzle with Greek dressing.

<u>Prep Time</u>: 25 minutes

<u>Nutritional Information</u>: Low in carbs, high in protein

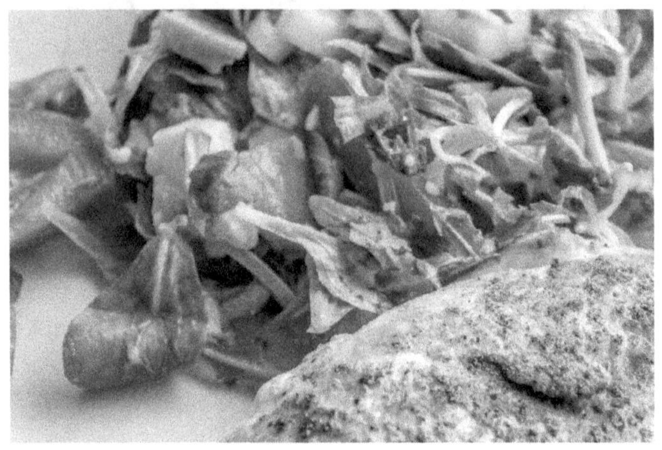

Turkey and Cranberry Salad:

<u>Ingredients</u>:

- Turkey breast
- Mixed greens
- Cranberries
- Almonds
- Balsamic vinaigrette

Instructions:

- Roast the turkey and mix it with greens.
- Add cranberries to it and use almonds as toppings.
- Finish it off with a vinaigrette as dressing.

Prep Time: 25 minutes

Nutritional Information: Low in carbs and rich in lean protein

Spinach and Strawberry Salad:

Ingredients:

- Fresh spinach
- Strawberries
- Goat cheese
- Almonds
- Balsamic reduction

Instructions:

- Toss the spinach with strawberries.

- Add the goat cheese and almonds as toppings then sprinkle with balsamic reduction.

<u>Prep Time</u>: 15 minutes

<u>Nutritional Information</u>: Low in carbs and high in vitamins

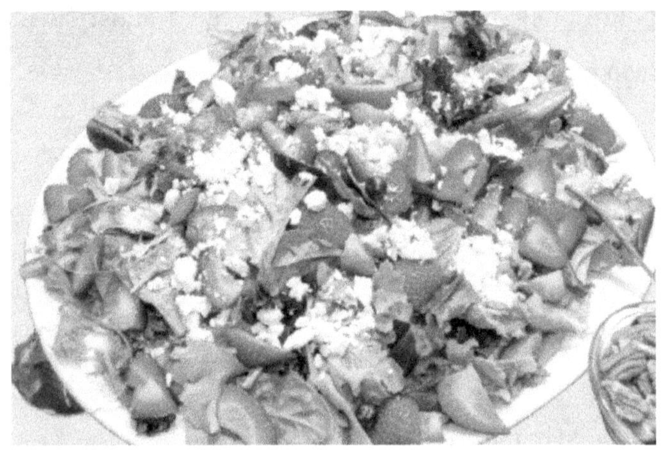

Cabbage and Apple Slaw:

<u>Ingredients</u>:

- Shredded cabbage
- Apples
- Walnuts

* Greek yogurt coleslaw dressing

Instructions:

* Mix the cabbage, apples, and walnuts together then stir with Greek yogurt coleslaw dressing.

Prep Time: 20 minutes

Nutritional Information: Low in carbs and high in fiber

Tuna and Chickpea Salad:

Ingredients:

* Canned tuna
* Chickpeas
* Cherry tomatoes
* Cucumber
* Lemon-tahini dressing

Instructions:

* Mix the tuna, chickpeas, tomatoes, and cucumber together.
* Garnish with lemon-tahini dressing.

<u>Prep Time</u>: 20 minutes

<u>Nutritional Information</u>: High in protein and moderate in carbs

Caprese Salad with Balsamic Glaze:

<u>Ingredients</u>:

- Fresh mozzarella
- Tomatoes
- Basil
- Balsamic glaze

<u>Instructions</u>:

- Arrange the mozzarella, tomatoes, and basil, then drizzle with balsamic glaze.

<u>Prep Time</u>: 15 minutes

<u>Nutritional Information</u>: Low in carbs and moderate in protein

CHAPTER 8: MEAL PLANS

This is a general meal plan for those with type 2 diabetes that does not take any other unique medical conditions or allergies into account. Individual nutritional requirements vary; thus, patients should consult a healthcare practitioner before making any dietary modifications. The nutritional information presented is based on basic guidelines and may not be applicable to everyone. It is not a substitute for expert medical advice, diagnosis, or treatment; it is only to assist in meal suggestions.

Day 1:

Breakfast: Greek yogurt parfait

Lunch: Grilled chicken salad

Dinner: Baked Salmon with Asparagus

Day 2:

Breakfast: Oatmeal with Berries and Nuts

Lunch: Quinoa and black bean bowl

Dinner: Sesame Ginger Tofu Stir-Fry

Day 3:

Breakfast: Whole-grain toast with smashed avocado

Lunch: Lentil and vegetable soup

Dinner: Turkey and Sweet Potato Hash

Day 4:

Breakfast: Low-carb smoothie

Lunch: Turkey and avocado wrap

Dinner: Quinoa and vegetable stir-fry

Day 5:

Breakfast: Cottage cheese and berry bowl

Lunch: Salmon and spinach salad

Dinner: Baked cod with lemon and herbs

Day 6:

Breakfast: Egg and Veggie Breakfast Wrap

Lunch: Chickpea and vegetable curry

Dinner: Turkey and vegetable skewers

Day 7:

Breakfast: Chia seed pudding

Lunch: Caprese salad with grilled chicken

Dinner: Grilled Lemon Herb Chicken

Day 8:

Breakfast: Sausage and Kale Breakfast Casserole

Lunch: Turkey and Bean Chili

Dinner: Grilled Chicken and Avocado Salad

Day 9:

Breakfast: Veggie omelet

Lunch: Tuna and avocado salad

Dinner: Cabbage and turkey sauté

Day 10:

Breakfast: Blueberry Almond Overnight Oats

Lunch: Eggplant and Chickpea Stew

Dinner: Lemon Garlic Shrimp with Zoodles

Day 11:

Breakfast: Almond flour pancakes

Lunch: Mediterranean Chickpea Salad

Dinner: Black Bean and Vegetable Quesadillas

Day 12:

Breakfast: Mango Tango Smoothie

Lunch: Mediterranean Quinoa salad

Dinner: Cauliflower Rice Stir-Fry

Day 13:

Breakfast: Turmeric and Veggie Scramble

Lunch: Quinoa Stuffed Bell Peppers

Dinner: Grilled Veggie and Chicken Kabobs

Day 14:

Breakfast: Cottage Cheese and Berry Stuffed Crepes

Lunch: Veggie and Turkey Stuffed Pepper

Dinner: Salmon and Cucumber Roll-Ups

Day 15:

Breakfast: Whole Grain Toast with Avocado

Lunch: Roasted Chickpeas

Dinner: Spinach and Mushroom Stuffed Chicken

Day 16:

Breakfast: Chocolate protein smoothie

Lunch: Caprese Salad with Balsamic Glaze

Dinner: Spaghetti Squash with Turkey Meatballs

Day 17:

Breakfast: Apple Cinnamon Chia Pudding

Lunch: Shirataki Noodle Stir-Fry with Tofu

Dinner: Broccoli and Chicken Skillet

Day 18:

Breakfast: Tomato and Basil Avocado Toast

Lunch: Vegetable Stir-Fry with Tofu

Dinner: Greek Chicken Skewers

Day 19:

Breakfast: Ricotta and Berry-stuffed French Toast

Lunch: Stuffed Bell Peppers with Turkey and Quinoa

Dinner: Zucchini Noodles with Turkey Bolognese

Day 20:

Breakfast: Peanut Butter Banana Toast

Lunch: Greek Salad with Chicken

Dinner: Shrimp and Broccoli Stir-Fry

Day 21:

Breakfast: Pesto and Tomato Egg Muffins

Lunch: Broccoli and Chicken Alfredo with Brown Rice Pasta

Dinner: Tuna Salad Lettuce Wraps

Day 22:

Breakfast: Salmon and Cream Cheese Stuffed Avocado

Lunch: Mushroom and Spinach Omelet

Dinner: Turkey and Cranberry Salad

Day 23:

Breakfast: Berry Bliss Smoothie

Lunch: Cabbage and Apple Slaw

Dinner: Turkey and Vegetable Skewers

Day 24:

Breakfast: Mediterranean Breakfast Bowl

Lunch: Sesame Ginger Beef Stir-Fry

Dinner: Turkey and Sweet Potato Hash

Day 25:

Breakfast: Almond and Berry Yogurt Parfait

Lunch: Dark Chocolate-Dipped Strawberries

Dinner: Cabbage and turkey sauté

Day 26:

Breakfast: Smoked Salmon and Cream Cheese Bagel

Lunch: Chickpea and Vegetable Curry

Dinner: Shrimp and Asparagus Salad

Day 27:

Breakfast: Cinnamon Apple Delight

Lunch: Greek Yogurt with Nuts and Berries

Dinner: Spaghetti Squash with Turkey Meatballs

Day 28:

Breakfast: Almond Flour Pancakes

Lunch: Lentil and vegetable soup

Dinner: Chicken and Vegetable Curry

Finish your meal with a favorite dessert. You can also have snacks with smoothies, but keep track of your intake.

CONCLUSION

This type 2 diabetes cookbook seeks to provide people with a practical and entertaining way to manage their health via mindful eating. The path to optimal health entails not only limitation, but also an enjoyment of diverse, tasty, and nutrient-dense meals. Individuals with type 2 diabetes can improve their general well-being by eating a well-balanced diet that promotes stable blood sugar levels and weight management.

Throughout this cookbook, we have attempted to give a varied selection of recipes that cater to a variety of tastes, dietary requirements, and lifestyles. From hearty breakfasts to filling dinners and delectable snacks, each meal is carefully designed to minimize the impact on blood sugar. The cookbook's emphasis on complete, unprocessed products, lean meats, and complex carbohydrates demonstrates its commitment to promoting a healthy and enjoyable way of eating.

Adding these meals to your daily routine does more than only manage type 2 diabetes; it also fosters a positive relationship with food. We encourage you to experiment with flavors, adapt recipes to your preferences, and find joy in making meals that benefit your entire health.

Remember that this cookbook is not a rigorous rulebook, but rather a guide to make informed decisions that are consistent with your health goals. It is about developing habits that promote your well-being and realizing that tiny, consistent changes can result in major benefits.

As you embark on this culinary journey, we recommend that you engage with healthcare specialists or registered dietitians to customize these dishes to your unique needs. Your health is unique, and expert advice can help you navigate the complexities of properly managing type 2 diabetes.